Psychosocial Care
of Cancer Survivors

Psychosocial Care of Cancer Survivors

A Clinician's Guide and Workbook
for Providing Wholehearted Care

CHERYL KRAUTER, MFT

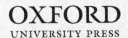

OXFORD
UNIVERSITY PRESS

OXFORD
UNIVERSITY PRESS

Oxford University Press is a department of the University of Oxford. It furthers
the University's objective of excellence in research, scholarship, and education
by publishing worldwide. Oxford is a registered trade mark of Oxford University
Press in the UK and certain other countries.

Published in the United States of America by Oxford University Press
198 Madison Avenue, New York, NY 10016, United States of America.

Library of Congress Cataloging-in-Publication Data
Names: Krauter, Cheryl, author.
Title: Psychosocial care of cancer survivors : a clinician's guide
and workbook for providing wholehearted care / Cheryl Krauter.
Description: New York, NY : Oxford University Press, [2018] |
Includes bibliographical references.
Identifiers: LCCN 2018010772 | ISBN 9780190636364 (pbk.)
Subjects: | MESH: Cancer Survivors—psychology | Survivorship | Psychotherapy—methods |
Existentialism—psychology | Humanism | Interpersonal Relations
Classification: LCC RC271.M4 | NLM QZ 260 | DDC 616.99/40651—dc23
LC record available at https://lccn.loc.gov/2018010772

9 8 7 6 5 4 3 2 1

Printed by Webcom, Inc., Canada

everything here
seems to need us

—Rainer Maria Rilke

Contents

Who is a cancer survivor? In the quest to take cancer out of the closet, so to speak, the term is ever present, on billboards and on websites. If you peruse the most widely used lay cancer sites online (American Cancer Society, American Society of Clinical Oncology, National Coalition for Cancer Survivorship), you might conclude that anyone who has ever heard the word *cancer* might be considered a survivor. In my work and in this book, the term *survivor* refers to those who have completed treatment for cancer, are disease-free and are attempting to revise their lives while adjusting to their changed post-treatment emotional and physical state.

The importance to survivors of a landing place following their discharge from being a cancer patient cannot be overstated. I have heard many survivors say that the worst day of their lives was not the day they received their cancer diagnosis, but the day they finished treatment. During the months of therapy, their oncology team has told them—day by day, hour by hour—what to do and how to do it. Everything from diet to skin care has been covered by a nurse, a booklet, or a handout. There was nothing left to the imagination. There was a plan and no wavering from the plan. Now that they are disease-free, how will they know if they are having a headache or cancer has reemerged as a brain tumor? Is the extreme fatigue experience normal, or there is another comorbid disease or aftereffect of treatment rearing its ugly head? The questions go on and on and on. Survivors are always waiting for the next test result, the next scan to find out the state of their health. The ability to trust one's body and its signals vanishes with the initial diagnosis of cancer.

How does a survivor gain the understanding that the post-treatment phase of cancer is not the result of the flick of a switch, restoring their former healthy self? How does one identify resources that are needed to continue their personal healing process? This is the puzzle that survivorship programs are assigned to solve. Cheryl Krauter and I are united in our quest to bring the post-treatment phase of cancer care into the light. It has been a grave disservice to those who may not have a background in healthcare or a provider who can review their current symptoms in relation to the treatment and experience they have had and make referrals and recommendations. Ms. Krauter's book for survivors, *Surviving the Storm* (New York: Oxford University Press, 2017), has empowered people to take on the management of their post-treatment selves. All aspects of life after cancer cure are covered therein in an accessible and honest approach, including creating one's own very personal care plan. The notion that support is needed during the period once treatment is finished should be raised by the clinical team and not relegated to a status of secrecy. By doing your patients the favor of imparting this information to them, you are providing truly patient-centered care that enables them to act instead of continuing in a state of trauma.

If you are an oncologist, your patients and many of your colleagues and staff consider you to be a hero. You cure cancer. You understand the way cancer sneaks around the body and attacks organs and lymph systems. You know the combination of drugs, surgery, or radiation therapy that you predict will eradicate cancer and set the person right. So it should not be a surprise that your patients want to be grateful and healthy when they see you for follow-up care. They want to honor the curative effect that you have had on their lives and not trouble you with the fact that they still cannot seem to sleep through the night, which is affecting their work and family life. Besides, they do not want to waste the short amount of time that they have with you during a follow-up appointment. They want to bask in their success in beating cancer with the one they feel is responsible and not subject you to a laundry list of physical and emotional complaints. During treatment, they have acted as though they were who they thought themselves to be. Now, they are confronting who they have become. It is up to you to ask the questions that elicit the truth about their current state and to provide resources that will support their quest for wellness. Your patients are unable or unwilling to ruin the mood of cure. Their post-treatment lives are once again in your hands, waiting for you to inquire of their current state of well-being, listen generously, and discuss potential healing mechanisms.

You, as their trusted clinician, can make a difference in the lives of cancer survivors. By reading this book and utilizing the tools and recommendations that Cheryl provides, you will begin to see the ways that you can deliver value by providing care that is supportive of and desperately needed by this group. We are not demanding that you keep current with the myriad services available in your community aimed at survivors, but that you have someone within your cancer center or clinic that has the expertise and that you know how to get patients that resource information. Referral to a post-treatment clinician such as a nurse practitioner or nurse navigator can provide expert direction and valuable support for your patients without detracting from the follow-up care that you will continue to provide.

We are counting on you, Ms. Krauter and I. We want to see you take a leadership role within your practice, within your specialty, with primary care providers that your patients have returned to. Think outside the Commission on Cancer mandate to provide a treatment summary and care plan documents to all survivors. Don't fall into the trap of checking the box and considering it done. Do it because it is the ethical and right thing for your patients.

I would be remiss if I didn't remind you to institute wholehearted care for yourself. How do you maintain passion for your work and avoid burnout? This is easier said than done, I know, but vital to your well-being. I encourage you to consider your whole heart and think about what nourishes your soul and stimulates your curiosity, wonder, sense of humor, and inquisitiveness. Take action and make a commitment to taking care of you. Bringing your best self to work not only supports you, but also is reflected in the care of your patients.

Meridithe A. Mendelsohn, MPA, PhD
Program Manager, Cancer Survivorship
Swedish Cancer Institute
Seattle, Washington

Prologue

The end of cancer treatment is only the beginning of the story of cancer survivorship. As more people survive cancer, there is a growing need for healthcare clinicians of all disciplines to attend to the post-treatment needs of cancer patients, to acknowledge the distress of their partners and family members, and to recognize the concerns of formal and informal caregivers. This expanding territory of cancer survivorship care extends beyond the oncology setting as survivors deal with numerous physical and psychosocial issues that follow them for the rest of their lives. Given this reality, the material in this book is presented as appropriate and relevant for all healthcare clinicians who are among those professionals who serve cancer survivors, people living with cancer, and their loved ones.

My goal with *Psychosocial Care of Cancer Survivors: A Clinician's Guide and Workbook for Providing Wholehearted Care* is to address the treatment needs of individual patients who are cancer survivors, as well as focus on the both the education and the needs of clinicians who work with them. The healing relationship requires that we to come to our work with an engaged, wholehearted stance and understand that it is within relationship that the deepest healing occurs. Throughout this book, patient-centered care is defined as person-centered care, which is essentially the definition of the healing relationship. Therefore, this book focuses on humanizing patient care as well as the necessity of clinician self-care, collegial collaboration, and the importance of a personal and professional commitment to lifelong learning. As clinicians, we cannot be present with our patients if we are not present with ourselves. This humanistic perspective is valuable to students who are entering the healthcare field because, as beginning clinicians, they have the opportunity to change and humanize a distressed healthcare system.

The healing relationship cannot be quantified because we are not in relationship with a statistic. It is not possible to measure the distress of the human heart by using a mathematical formula, and each individual's story is unique regardless of the common threads that can be identified and traced to the larger population. Because quality of care cannot always be accurately measured, we are called on to trust and value what we cannot always quantify. While statistics are important when it comes to research, the National Cancer Institute reported that "statistical trends are not usually applicable to individual patients." So, while it's clear that there's a need for competent, evidence-based research to fund programs that address the impact and the challenges of cancer and provide funds for research, the need for quality emotional care for the physical, emotional, and psychic trauma that is carried by cancer survivors must be equally validated. Alongside the importance of person-centered care for patients is the need to attend to the concerns of healthcare clinicians in regard not only to their survival in a highly stressful field but also to the advocacy for their professional growth and the support of the significance of personal meaning in the work that they have been called to do.

This book is presented in two parts. Part I of *Psychosocial Care of Cancer Survivors* focuses on skillful means for providing humanistic patient care, while Part II presents material designed to offer clinicians pragmatic structures to help with the implementation of methods for relational patient treatment as well as provide a framework that benefits them both personally and professionally. Written from the perspective of a clinician–survivor, this book is about the healing power of relationship for both patient and practitioner as they negotiate the complex world of cancer survivorship.

Acknowledgments

I am grateful to Andrea Knobloch at Oxford University Press for her caring support and for being an invaluable advocate of my work.

Thank you to Allison Applebaum, PhD, for her collegial support and friendship.

My appreciation goes to Meridithe Mendelsohn, PhD, for the supportive and inspiring conversations we began in 2009 involving the important and necessary work of person-centered survivorship care. Our connection is representative of what can be truly meaningful in a collegial relationship.

I am grateful to be a part of the Women's Cancer Resource Center (WCRC) in Oakland, California, where I have been given the great privilege to work with a diverse population and become a lifelong learner in the principles of cultural humility. I would like to acknowledge the staff at WCRC, a beautiful, strong, intelligent, and caring group of women whose dedication to attending to the underserved population is the epitome of humanistic care.

Thank you to the clinicians who are an important part of my professional and personal support network: Elaine Cooper, PhD; Rose Phelps, MFT; Lois Friedlander, MFT; Mary Ann Kassier, LCSW; Orah Krug, PhD; Geraldine Alpert, PhD; Cheryl Jones, MFT; Joan Steidinger, PhD, and Randy Dunagan, MFT.

A special shout out to James Fishman, LCSW, for being a creative and inspiring colleague and a dear friend.

Thank you to my clients, students, trainees, and interns who have honored me with their trust and courageously shared their lives. I hope I have adequately expressed all that you have given to me over the years.

I dedicate the thoughts and theories in *Psychosocial Care of Cancer Survivors* to my mentor, James F. T. Bugental, PhD, and to the teacher who was my first inspiration as a psychotherapist, Carl A. Faber, PhD. I keep both of them in the room with me at all times.

With deep gratitude to Brooke Warner of Warner Coaching and She Writes Press, whose wise guidance and collaboration is valuable beyond words. Her questions and comments sharpened my writing and brought clarity to the material being presented while also making me a better clinician. Thanks, Brooke, for being such an integral part of this project.

This book was written during the most challenging year of my life as I dealt with the grief of the sudden loss of my husband in May 2016. I feel a deep appreciation to Wilma Friesema and Diane Gravenites for being by my side as I negotiated the turbulent seas of loss. I am grateful for the loving support of Bonnie Fluke, Bill and Shash Woods, Paul Cameron, Georgia Stathis, Diana Lovett, Steve Lipson, Richard Heasley, Leslie Weir, Barbara and Peter Sapienza, Tony and Cathi Christo, Cathy and Dale Thorne, and the wonderful folks in my neighborhood.

Words cannot adequately express my deep gratitude and love for my consultation group and dear friends Chris Armstrong, Sandra Bryson, and Lou Dangles for always holding me close and having my back every step of the way. I really could not have stayed on my feet without you.

And, of course, with love to my son, Ben, for being a bright light in my life.

Introduction

Hospital Writing Workshop
Arriving late, my clinic having run
past 6 again, I realize I don't
have cancer, don't have HIV, like them,
these students who are patients, who I lead
in writing exercises, reading poems.
For them, this isn't academic, it's
reality: I ask that they describe
an object right in front of them, to make
it come alive, and one writes about death,
her death, as if by just imagining
the softness of its skin, its panting rush
into her lap, that she might tame it; one
observes instead the love he lost, he's there,
beside him in his gown and wheelchair,
together finally again. I take
a good, long breath; we're quiet as newborns.
The little conference room grows warm, and right
before my eyes, I see that what I thought
unspeakable was more than this, was hope.

—Rafael Campo, MD[1]

The closer I get to the entrance of the breast health center, the more I experience fear. The energy of fear in the beautifully decorated hallway is so strong that it seeps into my pores, quickens my heartbeat, and shortens my breath. After nearly a decade and all the tests and scans, some bringing bad news, most delivering the welcome "all clear," I remind myself to breathe.

The unspeakable suffering of illness sits in the examining rooms, the hospital operating rooms, and countless waiting rooms in cancer clinics and oncology offices across the country. And then, once the storms of cancer are quieted, the months and, it is hoped, years of living with cancer—or being in the uncertainty of remission—can be confusing and disorienting and can involve suffering that too often goes unacknowledged and neglected. Cancer survivorship is not romantic, and it does not have a predictable end point. However, the challenging realities of survivorship can be addressed and softened with a humanistic perspective that offers both growth and solace as people move forward in their lives.

I began my career as a psychotherapist, and then later, after my own journey through cancer, I shifted my concentration to help cancer survivors move through their experience with cancer to a place of healing and growth. As a humanistic psychotherapist in practice for over thirty-five years, I never anticipated that I would come from a personal experience with cancer to work with those whose lives have been impacted by a cancer diagnosis. I consider myself a "survivor provider" and I call the work I do with cancer survivors "the specialty that chose me." As I sit with people whose lives have been affected by a cancer diagnosis, I am reminded of what an honor it is to work with them as they courageously find their way through struggles and triumphs.

The healing relationship is at the core of the commitment that is made when a person enters the helping profession. It is the relationship between human beings that makes working in cancer healthcare meaningful. Yet many clinicians face a disturbing lack of personal connection, loss of meaning, isolation, and numerous other difficulties working within the current cancer healthcare system. As a psychotherapist, 99% of my work happens within the relationship between my client and me. Without that bond and a strong level of trust, we cannot travel together down bumpy roads. Currently, we in the healing profession are in danger of forgetting or losing that sense that *we* are part of a relationship, and that our needs and wants are also involved. Those of us who are the caregivers are hurting. As we take care of others, we struggle to take care of ourselves. We are left to quietly cope with our own pain, stress, and struggles with burnout, often feeling alone in a system that is overloaded and underfunded. Integrative care that pays attention to the whole person is becoming more of a focus in the care of patients. Why not also for the providers?

This book is for those of you who make a difference every day in the lives of people who are struggling with a diagnosis of cancer—you who work long into the night when others have gone home in order to care for those who are in distress. Working in the cancer healthcare system isn't just a job, it's a life commitment and a calling. Remember when you decided to work in the healing profession? The essence of that choice was likely a desire to be of service to those who are suffering, to move beyond the boundaries of your personal world and enter a community whose commitment is to help others. There was likely a desire to form relationships that offered both you and your patients a meaningful collaboration based on healing.

On June 3, 2014, the *Los Angeles Times* reported, "As of January 1, there were nearly 14.5 million people alive in the United States who had been diagnosed with some type of cancer. By 2024, that figure is projected to reach 18.9 million, according to a report released this week by the American Cancer Society."[2]

These numbers herald the good news that cancer is no longer assumed to be a death sentence. But as more people are successfully treated and survive a cancer diagnosis, there is an increased demand on clinicians to assist in helping them to negotiate the post-treatment world as cancer survivors. There is also a need for attention for those who may not be cancer-free but are able to go on with their lives as people living with cancer. And we must include the partners and the families, as cancer affects all of those who are related to the patient. Survivors, their partners, and their families all need help in navigating the uncertainties and concerns of their future. These growing numbers affect today's world of post-treatment cancer care, and as clinicians we are struggling to survive the storm of cancer without becoming numb and losing touch with what it means to offer cancer survivors, their partners, and their families authentic emotional healing from their experiences with a cancer diagnosis.

Psychosocial Care of Cancer Survivors: A Clinician's Guide and Workbook for Providing Wholehearted Care presents a humanistic alternative to the existing cancer survivorship care plan requirement. Written from the perspective of humanistic existential psychology, this text covers the theoretical foundation of humanistic psychotherapy, which adopts a holistic approach to human existence and pays special attention to such phenomena as creativity, free will, and positive human potential. This approach allows the merging of mindfulness and cognitive therapy while offering pragmatic examples, structures, and tools that support providers in the use of an integrative and relational approach in their work with cancer survivors and their communities.

This companion volume to *Surviving the Storm: A Workbook for Telling Your Cancer Story* (New York: Oxford University Press, 2017), a workbook written for cancer survivors, their partners, and their families, is for healthcare professionals working with the psychosocial and emotional concerns of cancer survivors. This includes oncologists, surgeons, primary-care physicians, psychologists, psychiatrists, nurses, physician assistants, social workers, and psychotherapists working in private practice who provide valuable services to this community. This workbook is intended not only to assist in our work with our patients, but also to open a conversation between those of us who work in cancer healthcare. We can create a dialogue that addresses how we can find a deeper sense of satisfaction by bringing our humanity to our work.

PART I—The Humanistic Approach: Changing the Way We Do Patient Care

There has been much discussion and debate on how to implement patient-centered care in cancer survivorship. Concerns about cost-effectiveness, limited resources in an overcrowded healthcare system, and clinicians who are overscheduled and overworked all contribute to a belief that we don't have the capacity to humanize care for the whole person. This belief negates the power of human connection as bedrock in a healing relationship. The challenge is not lack of time or funds, but rather finding a path that returns us to this basic and universal foundation of human contact. We need to have a conversation of change.

Humanistic existential psychotherapy, which focuses on the whole person and the person's potential and natural drive toward authenticity, is an excellent match for quality survivorship care in that it offers both patient and providers a way to connect in a relational manner. This contemplative perspective emphasizes shared human needs such as love, belonging, and personal meaning and expands beyond the learning-based behavioral and psychosocial resources that are currently available to cancer patients and their families. It provides options that differ from the support group and medical models of treatment, opening up an alternative to the mode of managing or tolerating the issues of cancer into the realm of awareness, exploration, acceptance, and transformation. While it is tempting to find solutions that try to "fix a problem," there is much to be gained from learning how to live with uncertainty and from delving more deeply into the emotional residue of cancer. There is no cure for cancer, yet some people may experience a disease-free remission, while others continue to live for the rest of their remaining life in some type of cancer treatment. Regardless of diagnosis or prognosis, the opportunity for healing is present. Healing isn't always about a cure or getting better, but it can occur in deep, surprising, and unexpected ways. This framework holds that healing is possible even when there is no cure for illness, and as such it is applicable for clinicians who are helping cancer patients and their families learn to deal with the uncertainties of a cancer diagnosis, especially as these people move into the post-treatment period.

As cancer patients enter the post-treatment phase of their lives, they can benefit from being helped to free themselves from fearful assumptions surrounding their survival and to let go of beliefs that hold them back from living as fully as possible, regardless of whatever prognosis they have been given. Awareness and growth can occur in surprising and illuminating ways even in times of despair and darkness. Both the provider and the patient are served when we bring this openness and trust to the consulting rooms, the hospitals, and the cancer clinics.

The existential framework holds that the core issues we face as human beings are anxiety, loneliness, isolation, despair, and ultimately death. This perspective acknowledges the lack of control inherent in existence, that we are limited creatures who suffer inevitable losses in our lives. We do not live in a controlled environment of our own making (although most of us attempt to refute this impossibility in a multitude of creative endeavors), and we are especially reminded of the contingencies of our lives through a life-threatening illness such as cancer.

While we are impacted by biology, circumstances, culture, and environment, we still have choices in how we respond to these unexpected twists and turns of our lives. The existential perspective poses that difficulties arise when we forget that we have choice as well as the capacity to find meaning in our lives regardless of our circumstances. It doesn't say that choices are always black or white, right or wrong, or even good or bad. Sometimes, choices involve deciding on the best possible outcome that you can expect when you are in a terrible predicament. This perspective is especially poignant for those living with cancer. There are times when we simply have to make "good enough" choices. In their book, *Existential Humanistic Therapy*, Kirk J. Schneider and Orah T. Krug wrote, "Existential therapy is about helping people to reclaim and reown their lives."[3] *Psychosocial Care of Cancer Survivors* applies this basic tenet to work with survivors as they negotiate the space between being a cancer patient and becoming a cancer survivor.

The Importance of Caring

The care of patients is the most important and demanding work of the clinician, regardless of the clinician's discipline. Integrating mindfulness, personal development, and effective communication skills into the repertoire of the healthcare provider addresses the building of this core aspect of the healing relationship. It has been shown that there are significant benefits to teaching cancer healthcare providers communication skills as it builds confidence and comfort in responding to the emotional needs of the patient. Beyond this basic level of communication, clinicians can learn to develop an empathic alliance with their patients that includes listening, respect, honesty, openness, and compassion. But what does it mean to develop an alliance with your patients, and what are the qualities of an authentic relationship with another human being? *Psychosocial Care of Cancer Survivors* will help you explore what it means to create an authentic connection that sets the tone for collaborative and meaningful relationships in your work with cancer survivors. As you explore your own personal choices regarding the healing relationship, you learn what works and what doesn't work and find ways to balance your personal and professional life.

As clinicians, we can learn a great deal about our patients by listening to them. Like drawing a perfect circle, however, this is often easier proposed than executed. Time constraints wreak havoc with a more personal touch, but we can no longer use this as an excuse for not paying better attention to the people we serve. A thorough method of distress screening needs to be used to determine the concerns of people post-treatment. We need to identify resources and make appropriate referrals to services for our patients. Current distress screening tools are adequate only in their assessment of needs, not in the attention to those needs. The small boxes we provide for patients to check do not fully cover or address emotions that cannot be reduced to one word or that cannot be easily described or defined. Distress screening is a pathway to identify what a patient needs so that the patient may be referred to resources that can provide assistance. It can show the territory where the patient is traveling, but then it needs to provide a path offering resources and referrals. Basically, simple distress screening is a listening tool, and, in that way, it guides both the patient and the provider in naming the challenges that are present. Yet, all too often, these short screening forms are merely filed and forgotten, leaving the patient in unattended distress. It is unethical to identify emotional difficulties and trauma and then not offer assistance. Clearly, this system needs a "refresh."

When we really listen to others, we hear not only the words they speak but also that which is not being spoken, and this helps us to begin to know the whole person. We watch how they move, we look in their eyes and become aware of what we see there, we notice their sighs and the times when there is a catch in their voice. We hear the inflections in their voice and see how they clutch their hands or pick at their fingers. We can learn from the words they use as well as from the expressions on their face. We know others and are known when we allow ourselves to touch each other, and it is these small moments of contact that connect us and create an authentic alliance that builds the healing relationship.

Healing and transforming things can happen between people when there is the true presence of mutual openness to the wind. Listeners that have brought themselves to this mystery time and time again become deeply wise and powerful people. Awed by their participation, they become better and better listeners. Their souls are weathered souls which carry not only their own life wounds, but those of friends and lovers. Some rare listeners seem to feel the wounds of the world.

—Carl A. Faber, PhD, *On Listening*[4]

"When I used to see a patient who'd been admitted to the emergency room," (the medical specialist) said, "I would read an account of what the patient had said and done and what the doctor thought. Now what I get are the results of tests. I used to have a story, an understanding. Sometimes I can't figure out what happened to the patient. I think medicine has lost its narrative."

—Nora Gallagher, *The Sun Magazine*[5]

Listening to someone tell you their story is a privilege. In my book, *Surviving the Storm,* people are given a structure to explore and express the stories of their experiences with a cancer diagnosis. *Psychosocial Care of Cancer Survivors: A Clinician's Guide and Workbook for Providing Wholehearted Care* is a guide for clinicians designed to assist you in helping your patients embark into the post-treatment phase. I have come to believe that the essential aspect of moving into survivorship in an integrated and holistic way is for all those involved to have the chance to tell their stories and to explore their inner world within an existential humanistic framework that integrates emotional care into the physical and behavioral aspects of survivorship. Information is helpful but only carries us so far in the facilitation of personalized healing. In all the cancer-themed talks, workshops, and events I have attended, as well as those where I have presented, I have witnessed the great need survivors have to speak about their experience. I've watched eyes glaze over as another expert talks and have looked into the faces of fear and distress as people sit silently with no avenue of expression. And then, when it's time for questions and comments, people burst out of their seats, eagerly speaking the stories of what has happened for them. When I interviewed cancer survivor Pam T., she told me, "Completing treatment doesn't close the door on that chapter of your life; you can't just dust off your hands and be done with it. The emotional and physical trauma remains."

Many of the characteristics of existential humanistic therapy have been incorporated into other therapeutic approaches, such as narrative therapy. A narrative interview may be used as an alternative to a behavioral assessment to give the patient an opportunity to create or tell his or her story. Offering patients a workbook is another option that serves to support them in telling the stories of their experience. By giving them a structure designed to assist in personal expression, they both become the author of what's happened to them and have the chance to write what will come next. Using a narrative interview or giving people the structure to write their stories is a way to provide them with an avenue of expression for some of the suffering they have endured. By fostering this expression, clinicians can offer cancer survivors a way to begin to develop a sense of awareness of where they are now in their lives as well as aid them in discovering what they want as they move forward. Guiding your patients in a manner that goes beyond coping or managing uncertainty and helps them to move into an exploration of who they are at this juncture of their life deepens the process of looking at the emotional needs of cancer survivors.

PART II—Taking Care of Others and Ourselves: Methods of Humanistic Patient Care and a Guide to Clinician Self-Care

Portion of physicians entering US medical internships who suffer from depression: 1/30. Portion who suffer from depression at some point in their internship: 1/2.

—Sunbeams, *The Sun Magazine*[6]

Addressing issues of self-care and burnout in the healthcare profession is the second, if not equally important, theme in *Psychosocial Care of Cancer Survivors*. In 2012, an article written by the Mayo Group in the *Archives of Internal Medicine* showed that 46% of the 7,000 physicians surveyed felt at least one aspect of burnout. In December 2015, Medscape medical news reported that physician burnout has climbed by 10%, bringing the total to 55%. Burnout symptoms were identified as emotional exhaustion, depersonalization, and low sense of personal accomplishment. The relationship that we have with ourselves often becomes overlooked and even forgotten as we are continually challenged with serving the needs of others. There is no more painful abandonment than the abandonment of the self. And what is true is that we cannot be present for others when we have lost our connection with ourselves and what matters to us.

The providers of services to cancer patients and their families are not officially included in the current definition of cancer survivor. Yet survivors are doctors, nurses, social workers, and many others who work long hours (some doing more than three or four jobs) treating people who are struggling with this devastating disease alongside the patients. You are on the front lines day after day, night after night, battling not only illness but also antiquated structures and procedures that hamper your ability to perform the healing work you are committed to providing. You spend countless hours in front of a computer rather than in front of a person. You are constantly faced with the lack of money to provide services and adequate staffing. Your trauma does not have a beginning or end; you face emotional exhaustion on a consistent basis. Underneath your professional role as a clinician, you are a human being who also needs to pay attention to yourself as a whole person. These difficult issues of burnout were addressed in a piece in the *New York Times*, which included this statement: "'Doctors are losing their inspiration,' Dr. [Tait D.] Shanafelt said, 'and that is a very frightening thing.'"[7] It is extremely consequential and depressing when you lose the sense that what you are doing has meaning.

Self-care in the healing profession is essential not only for the longevity of the practitioner but also for the practitioner's quality of life. Quality of life is not exclusive to patient care. Work–life balance is a serious concern for clinicians. Attention to the high rate of burnout in healthcare providers is critical, and the awareness and subsequent attention to the balance of the professional and personal lives of clinicians who struggle with the heavy demands of their work is crucial. There is a need for an emphasis on self-care for the clinician that provides pragmatic structure and support designed to address the issues of burnout, meaningful communication, and personal and professional fulfillment.

No Matter What We Are Doing, We Are Working With People

Psychosocial Care of Cancer Survivors may be used as a clinical resource by healthcare practitioners with the goal of enhancing communication with both patients and colleagues. It addresses the questions of how to bring a humanistic approach and quality attention to the growing needs of patients in the post-treatment phase of a cancer diagnosis. Clinical skills, communication tools, and exercises are included for use by healthcare practitioners in order to provide useful practices and solutions regarding their involvement in survivorship care with the intention of increasing the efficacy and satisfaction of their work.

In the end, what people will remember is how well they were cared for. The patients will recall a compassionate touch and the ways in which they were seen and heard in moments of sorrow and celebration. Held in an honest atmosphere of respect and concern, they will feel grateful for being treated as a human being and not merely another invisible patient. The clinician's authentic and empathic manner of relating sets the tone for a collaborative and healing relationship.

A cancer diagnosis no longer means that someone will die. With the advances in medical treatment, people are now surviving or living with cancer when, in the past, they would have died. Better screening, sophisticated imaging tools, and educated information leading to a deeper and more thorough understanding of cancer have all allowed for more successful outcomes. However, an atmosphere of aliveness is often missing in the treatment of the person who has cancer. In the post-treatment phase of cancer, there can be a profound sense of isolation and disconnection as survivors are "unplugged" from their cancer healthcare team. Technology and knowledge have brought advances but at the same time created a mechanized system where people can feel dehumanized and marginalized. By bringing a humanistic attitude into cancer healthcare, we have a chance to initiate a subjective stance rather than remain in a system that objectifies both clinician and patient. Humanity in cancer care includes openness and humility and requires a commitment to self-awareness and the empathic understanding of others. Bringing our humanity to our work gives us the opportunity to arouse a feeling of inner healing power within ourselves and our patients.

Our power to heal is far less limited than our power to cure. Healing is not a relationship between an expert and a problem. . . . It is a relationship between human beings.

—Rachel Naomi Remen, MD[8]

Notes

1. Rafael Campo, MD, Hospital Writing Workshop, copyright © 2014 by Rafael Campo, *Comfort Measures Only: New and Selected Poems 1994–2016*, Duke University Press, Durham, NC, April 2018. This poem appeared in Poem-A-Day on January 3, 2014. https://www.poets.org/poetsorg/poem-day.

2. Karen Kaplan, Cancer Survivors in the US—14.5 Million Strong and Growing. *Los Angeles Times*, June 3, 2014.

3. Kirk J. Schneider and Orah T. Krug, *Existential–Humanistic Therapy*, American Psychological Association, Washington, DC, December 2010, p. 1.

4. Carl A. Faber, PhD, *On Listening*, Perseus Press, New York, NY, 1976, p. 20.

5. Nora Gallagher, Sunbeams. *The Sun Magazine*, January 2016. http://thesunmagazine.org/issues/481/sunbeams.

6. Excerpt from Sunbeams, *The Sun Magazine*, January 2016. http://thesunmagazine.org/issues/481. Quotation from *Harper's* Index, Archive/2015/November.

7. Pauline W. Chen, MD, The widespread problem of doctor burnout. *New York Times*, August 23, 2012.

8. Rachel Naomi Remen, MD, Some Thoughts on Healing. http://www.rachelremen.com/some-thoughts-on-healing. Published August 16, 2010.

PART I

The Humanistic Approach: Changing the Way We Do Patient Care

CHAPTER 1

Roots of Authenticity

The History and Foundation of Existential Humanistic Psychotherapy

You're on Earth. There's no cure for that.

—Samuel Beckett, *Endgame*[1]

In the fall of 1976, the doors to a new world opened, and I found myself entering a place with a labyrinth of dark passages and secret chambers filled with treasures. I had left my studies at a prestigious university in search of an authentic, humanistic psychology program and landed in a habitat of self-discovery known as the Humanistic Psychology Program or, as it was called, HPP. Innovators from the early days of humanistic psychology were core faculty, and, as students, we were fully engaged in an experiential process of clinical education. It was an exciting time as the field of psychology was changing from a behavioral, analytic viewpoint, moving away from a reductionistic view of human consciousness, and beginning to open to the myriad possibilities of growth inherent in the relationship between clinician and patient.

In the early days of psychology, we were taught to have rigid boundaries, keep ourselves separate, and avoid personal disclosure in a psychotherapy session. We trained rats, studied various psychopathologies, and then diagnosed human beings by what we had learned in books and scholarly papers. But then came the 1960s and the introduction of a new consciousness in the healing profession that involved letting go of pathologizing individuals and beginning to view them as whole human beings with a deep propensity for discovering and actualizing their inner potential. It was a wild and crazy time as old boundaries and ideologies fell apart, sometimes splitting at the seams in remarkable ways. The human potential movement was born.

Today in cancer healthcare, there is a poignant struggle to remain human and in contact with patients in ways that are meaningful. Uncertainty in the lives of cancer survivors and those who are living with cancer is the primary concern as they move forward in their lives. The emotional distress and trauma of a cancer diagnosis and its ensuing treatment are essential to address in quality survivorship care. Existential humanistic theory and practice have numerous applications in post-treatment cancer care as they attend to both individual and universal themes of what it means to be a human being who, while not having control of outcome, at least has choice.

The existential humanistic framework focuses on helping people free themselves from obsessive worries and scary stories by helping them to understand and work with the reality of living with uncertainty. Diseases cannot always be cured, events happen beyond our control, things change regardless of our plans—these are the conditions of existence, the basic fact of being alive. Cancer survivors who come face to face with these difficulties can be served by learning to explore and perhaps come to some sense of peace and acceptance of these realities. In editing their book, *Stories of the Spirit, Stories of the Heart,* Kornfield and Feldman wrote, "In times of such darkness we find ourselves longing for an ideal future or seeking miraculous formulas to protect us from pain and conflict. It is not easy for us to accept that there is no cure for living."[2]

In *The Search for Authenticity,* James F. T. Bugental wrote, "An existential orientation to personality and psychotherapy recognizes the human experience as the central face of existence, examines the vicissitudes of that experience in the perspective of the basic nature of being, and orients its growth-inducing efforts toward maximum accord with the whole of life."[3] This humanistic stance holds that people have an inherent capacity for aware and responsible self-direction and choice, and that the disconnection from an authentic self is the root of distress.

An existential perspective concentrates on helping a person discover meaning in a life in which we sometimes have to struggle with the choices we didn't put on our "to do" list. We mistakenly assume that there is always a good choice or a bad choice and that we must somehow find the good one to be "right." For those who have received a cancer diagnosis, the choices are often between the least horrific and the most horrific. The point is that even when it doesn't feel like it, we still have choice. Following a life-threatening event, such as a diagnosis of cancer, people can struggle with going forward in their lives, sometimes finding it difficult and confusing to know who they are and how to interact in their lives now that treatment has ended. They often experience themselves as deeply changed but have no structure to guide them in a deeper exploration of how they have been impacted by cancer.

An existential humanistic perspective provides a structure that can be adapted for survivors who are looking to reflect and explore themselves and their lives after cancer. The essential aims of this approach were described by Kirk Schneider and Orah Krug in their book *Existential Humanistic Therapy*, in which they wrote: "To summarize, E-H therapy has four essential aims: (a) to help clients become more present to themselves and others; (b) to help them experience the ways in which they can both mobilize and block themselves from fuller presence; (c) to help them take responsibility for construction of their current lives; and (d) to help them choose or actualize more expanded ways of being in their outside lives."[4]

The existential humanistic perspective integrates with other approaches to include a diverse array of therapeutic interventions to be used in working with cancer survivors. They are united by an emphasis on lived experience, authentic relationships, and acknowledgment of the subjective nature of human experience. Carl Rogers's client-centered therapy, also known as person-centered, nondirective, or Rogerian therapy, is one such counseling approach that requires the client to take an active role in his or her treatment, with the therapist being nondirective and supportive. In client-centered therapy, the client determines the course and direction of treatment, which speaks to the capacity of the patient to advocate for himself or herself when dealing with his or her medical treatment as well as survivorship care.

Client-centered therapy was developed in the 1940s and 1950s by the American psychologist Carl Rogers. Rogers was a humanistic psychologist who believed that how we live in the here and now and how our current perceptions affect us are more important than the past. He also believed that close personal relationships with a supportive environment of warmth, genuineness, and understanding are key for therapeutic change. Client-centered therapy differs from other forms of therapy largely because it does not focus on therapeutic techniques. What's most important instead is the quality of the relationship between the therapist and the client. This framework is readily translatable to patient-centered care in the cancer healthcare setting as it promotes a warm, caring connection between patient and provider. Indeed, putting the concept of "person-centered care" into practice humanizes care at all levels.

In the 1980s, Michael White and David Epstein developed what has come to be known as narrative therapy. Narrative therapy works from the proposition that there are alternative ways of making sense of our world, and that people can liberate themselves from old, problematic stories and create a story of their choice. Throughout life, personal experiences can be transformed into stories that are given meaning, which can help shape a person's understanding of who they are at a given moment in their lives. Like all humanistic therapies, narrative therapy is a collaborative and nonpathologizing approach to counseling that places each person in the position of being the expert of their own life, the author of their own story. In the face of life-threatening illness and its aftermath, the idea of hearing or telling stories as a way to heal may seem simplistic, yet the practice of storytelling is an ancient form that crosses class and culture as a way to connect and heal. Telling your story, being witnessed, and witnessing others can open up new realities and meaningful interactions that promote healing. Narrative therapy can be adapted in various, more conversational forms, such as narrative interview tools for clinicians, and also may be used to help survivors find a way to express themselves through a storytelling process. (See Krauter, *Surviving the Storm: A Workbook for Telling Your Cancer Story*, 2017.)

A Brief History of the Origins and Foundation of the Existential Humanistic Perspective

Existential-humanistic theory is rooted in the deepest recesses of recorded time. All who addressed the question of what it means to be fully and subjectively alive have partaken in the existential-humanistic quest. Existentialism derives from the Latin root ex-sistare, which literally means to "stand forth" or to "become" (May, 1958a, p. 12), whereas humanism originates in the ancient Greek tradition of "knowing thyself" (Grondin,

1995, p. 112). Therefore, existential humanism can be understood as a process of becoming and knowing oneself.

—Kirk J. Schneider and Orah Krug, *Existential Humanistic Psychotherapy*[5]

When I teach or weave academic material into an experiential group course, I often say that it is important to understand the roots of the work we are doing by having knowledge of its theoretical framework. This understanding provides the ground on which we stand when we are interacting with our clients or patients. As far back as 1928, Carl Jung wrote, "Learn your theories well but put them aside when you confront the mystery of the living soul."[6] So the majority of this book on the healing relationship focuses on the clinical applications of these theories. However, this chapter presents a brief background of existential humanistic thought and psychotherapy for a basic understanding of its history, values, and concepts. The Resources chapter provides titles for those who wish to read and study more about the background of existential humanism.

Existential humanism has its roots in phenomenological and existentialist thought that can be found in works by philosophical thinkers such as Martin Buber, Fyodor Dostoevsky, Viktor Frankl, Martin Heidegger, Edmund Husserl, Søren Kierkegaard, Friedrich Nietzsche, Jean-Paul Sartre, and Paul Tillich, among others. Taking form in mid–nineteenth-century Europe, existential philosophy revolved around concepts of freedom and responsibility. Existentialism grew out of a rebellion against a more dogmatic, linear, and prescribed way of being, and, to this day, the emphasis on authenticity and lived experience can be found in the theory and practice of current existential humanistic practice.

Kirk Schneider wrote, "In Kierkegaard's thesis, freedom emerges from crisis, and crisis from intellectual, emotional, or physical imprisonment."[7] Considering that a cancer diagnosis *is* a crisis based in reality, feeling stuck in the emotional distress associated with it can indeed feel like imprisonment. Following this thread, the use of an existential humanistic perspective in working with cancer survivors is beneficial in that it explicitly addresses the themes of uncertainty, isolation, and death, offering healing from the emotional distress of a life-threatening illness. In this manner, it suggests an alternative to the more behavioral approaches that are often utilized in the medical setting. In *The Search for Authenticity*, Bugental wrote that "the primary value of human life is to live in accord with (indeed, as part of) the ways things really are."[8] There are times when learning to live with "the way things really are" is the truth of what we have to work with, and in those moments we as human beings just have to stay with that. When we offer cancer survivors and those living with cancer the choice to explore themselves and embrace this truth—that sometimes it's just the way it is—we give them a way to free themselves so that they may fully engage in their lives regardless of their prognosis.

Moving forward into the twentieth century, existential thought appears in the work of those men who are considered to have laid the groundwork for humanistic psychology: William James, Otto Rank, Abraham Maslow, Carl Rogers, Rollo May, Erich Fromm, Clark Moustakas, Sidney Jourard, and James F. T. Bugental. Other innovators include Ludwig Binswanger and Henry Murray, both of whom based their work on the philosophy of Martin Heidegger and Edmund Husserl. Carl Gustav Jung's break from the psychoanalytic community allowed for his important contributions to the expanding field of psychology, which include a mythological and archetypal theoretical approach. Interestingly, existential thought was a form of protest toward behaviorism and Freudian psychoanalysis.

In 1943, Abraham Maslow developed a hierarchical theory of human motivation that proposed that people are motivated to achieve certain needs. When one need is fulfilled, people will move on to the next one, and so on. The earliest and most widespread version of Maslow's hierarchy of needs includes five motivational needs, often depicted as hierarchical levels within a pyramid. Those needs are basic physiological needs, safety, love and belonging, self-esteem, and self-actualization (Figure 1.1).

Physiological needs are mostly of a biological nature, air, food, drink, shelter, warmth, sleep, and sex. These basic needs must in some way be satisfactorily taken care of before someone has the capacity to move into a more introspective mode. Although this model appears linear, life experiences such as a cancer diagnosis may cause an individual to move up and down the pyramid depending on their needs during a particular

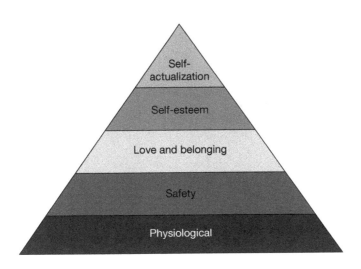

FIGURE 1.1

Maslow's hierarchy of needs.

period of their life. Some safety needs are closely related to physiological needs, such as protection, stability, security, order, and protection from elements (housing), but this level can begin to be more subjective in nature depending on the individual. As a person successfully negotiates a basic level of need, and once he or she achieves love and belonging, friendship, intimacy, and affection from his or her work group, family, and friends, then romantic relationships become significant in terms of personal happiness. Moving from the interpersonal, the inner personal needs of esteem, a sense of achievement and mastery, independence, and self-respect, as well as the respect of others, become the next layer of personal growth. The desired intention at the peak was deemed self-actualization, which means realizing personal potential, self-fulfillment, and seeking personal growth and peak experiences.

The next wave of change in the humanistic perspective arrived in the 1960s and was deemed the "human potential movement," which became synonymous with humanistic psychotherapies of that era. While the two are sometimes merged together, the strong base of humanistic psychology was the "third wave" or "third force" of psychology following psychoanalytic and behavioral modalities, and its founders were mostly psychologists rather than medical doctors, again separating the two fields of medicine and psychology. There was an emphasis on the value of group psychotherapy and a focus on including attention to a person's physical responses, thus initiating a holistic view of a mind and body connection that would later become the basis for somatic therapy. Again, the emphasis was moving away from a strict medical model and into a belief that a human being has within him or her the capacity for awareness and authentic growth. The focus shifted from a pathological view of humankind to assuming inherent health and the capacity for awareness. The use of the "here-and-now" process as an essential aspect of successful therapeutic change brought the clinician into the relationship with their patients, creating aliveness and depth. The humanistic approach considers human nature to be open-ended, flexible, and capable of an enormous range of experience. The person is viewed in a constant process of becoming, and psychotherapy as a process of allowing and fostering that becoming.

Humanism typically uses qualitative research methods, for example, personal journals, open-ended questionnaires, narrative interviews, and unstructured observations. However, it is difficult to place a more subjective study of human needs into an evidence-based category because of the core philosophy and bias toward a nonscientific view of humankind. Also, the areas investigated by humanism, such as consciousness and emotion, are difficult to study scientifically. However, qualitative research is useful for studies at the individual and group levels in that it can measure through a phenomenological process the ways in which people can feel supported, understood, and helped. Humanistic work opens up a space to affirm that another way to understand others is to sit down and talk with them, share their experiences, and be open to their feelings. The humanistic approach also helped to provide a more holistic view of human behavior, in contrast to the reductionist positions of scientific, behavioral, and traditional analytic approaches.

Humanistic psychology expanded its influence throughout the 1970s and the 1980s. Its impact can be understood in terms of three major areas:

1. It offered a new set of values for approaching an understanding of human nature and the human condition.
2. It offered an expanded horizon of methods of inquiry in the study of human behavior.

3. It offered a broader range of more effective methods in the professional practice of psychotherapy.[9]

Finally, existential humanistic psychology speaks to what it means to be human. Cancer and its aftermath bring us directly to our humanity in that we are faced with the one common denominator we all share: our mortality. Looking at and being with the common concerns, as well as the universal themes of life as a human being, are included in the humanistic perspective, which is why it is such a viable and valuable tool for serving the cancer survivor community.

It is not a case we are treating; it is a living, palpitating, alas, too often suffering fellow creature.

—John Brown, "Sunbeams"[10]

The Connection with Mindfulness

The connections between Eastern philosophy and humanistic psychology are visible in the ways that they explore and address similar concerns about the nature of human existence and consciousness. The current interest in including mindfulness practices in cancer healthcare has its basis in earlier humanistic and Eastern sources and seems a natural progression of humanism and client-centered and narrative work. In his book, *A Lamp in the Darkness,* Jack Kornfield wrote, "We all need healing at different times in our lives. At some point we need healing for physical illness. At other times we need to heal the trauma that we've suffered, and the ways to release the difficulties of the past we carry in our bodies."[11]

Martin Seligman is the founder of positive psychology, a field of study that examines healthy states, such as happiness, strength of character, and optimism. Psychology has traditionally focused on dysfunction—people with mental illness or other psychological problems—and how to treat it. Positive psychology, in contrast, is a relatively new field that examines how ordinary people can become happier and more fulfilled. While a positive outlook can encourage hope and well-being, it is equally important not to push this approach as what can be a support for some may be experienced as a pressure to be positive that can be oppressive for the cancer survivor.

Mindfulness programs in cancer care correspond to the humanistic approach. Take, for example, this definition of mindfulness used by the UCLA Center for Mindfulness:

Mindful awareness can be defined as paying attention to present moment experiences with openness, curiosity, and a willingness to be with what is. It is an excellent antidote to the stresses of modern times. It invites us to stop, breathe, observe, and connect with one's inner experience. There are many ways to bring mindfulness into one's life, such as meditation, yoga, art, or time in nature. Mindfulness can be trained systematically, and can be implemented in daily life, by people of any age, profession or background.[12]

While the essence of mindfulness parallels humanistic work, the difference can be seen in the statement that it can be "trained systematically," which speaks to a more pragmatic structure than is used in an existential humanistic approach. In this way, mindfulness can be viewed as a powerful companion to the existential humanistic process of personal exploration. Significant research has shown that the practice of mindfulness can be used to address health issues and boost the immune system; increase attention and focus; help with difficult mental states such as anxiety and depression, fostering well-being and less emotional reactivity; and thicken the brain in areas in charge of decision-making, emotional flexibility, and empathy. The current and ongoing investigations into the interactions between the brain and the body and the role of psychological well-being for health and recovery from illness are essential and indicate the usefulness of integrating this type of treatment into cancer survivorship programs as a way to promote healing and enhance well-being.

The Existential Humanistic Perspective in Survivorship Care

Our responsibility, in medicine, is to deal with human beings as they are.

—Atul Gawande, MD, *Being Mortal*[13]

Bringing an existential humanistic perspective into the work with cancer survivors is full of grit and grace. Beyond the philosophy and theory, we're talking about incorporating something into the real world where real people are suffering from pain, trauma, and emotional upheaval, which cannot be easily be measured or simply explained, much less healed. The value in incorporating the humanistic–existential psychotherapy framework into the cancer healthcare provider–patient relationship is that it offers a way to alleviate the suffering of those who have drawn the short straw of life-threatening illness as they face their uncertain futures. Oriented toward a compassionate, nonpathological frame that promotes acceptance, reflection, and relationship, this viewpoint suggests redefining professional competence as something that allows for compassionate engagement with patients, other professionals, and most important, oneself. The framework addresses living with uncertainty, the importance of quality relationships, and being present within yourself and with others and, in these ways, speaks to finding a strong way to provide quality care for cancer survivors, their partners, and their families.

In *Existential–Humanistic Therapy*, Schneider and Krug wrote: "The basic principles of existential therapy are an expansion on the basic principles of all therapies that point beyond the conventional emphasis on external, mechanical change. For example, existential therapy expands on medical intervention by inviting reflection on the meaning of the intervention."[14] The complexities of facing a life-threatening diagnosis are all too often overlooked in the limited time and space provided for the patient to actually absorb the news that they have been given. Using an inner search process to open up awareness and find a deeper, personal meaning in living with uncertainty in survivorship gives both provider and patient an opportunity to move beyond coping into an understanding of being fully alive. Introducing the patient to a way of life that can help them understand and accept what they are dealing with allows them to experience a stronger sense of personal power during a time when they feel helpless and without a sense of hope for their future.

In our work, we must remember that it doesn't take any more time to be human, it doesn't cost anything to have an authentic connection with others, and when we open up to the suffering of others, we are all healed.

Notes

1. Samuel Beckett, *Endgame*, Grove Press, New York, 1992; premiered April 3, 1957, Royal Court Theatre, London.
2. Jack Kornfield and Christina Feldman, editors, *Stories of the Spirit, Stories of the Heart: Parables of the Spiritual Path from Around the World*, Harper, San Francisco, 1991, p. 97.
3. James F. T. Bugental, PhD, *The Search for Authenticity*, Irvington, New York, 1981, p. 1.
4. Kirk J. Schneider and Orah Krug, *Existential–Humanistic Therapy*, American Psychological Association, Washington, DC, December 2010, p. 67.
5. Schneider and Krug, *Existential Humanistic Psychotherapy*, p. 5.
6. Carl Gustav Jung, *Contributions to Analytical Psychology*, Harcourt Brace, New York, 1928.
7. Kirk Schneider, Existential–Humanistic Theories, in *Essential Psychotherapies, Third Edition: Theory and Practice*, edited by Stanley B. Messer and Alan S. Gurman, Guilford Press, New York, 2011, p. 261.
8. Bugental, *Search for Authenticity*, p. 14.
9. S. A. McLeod, Humanism. *Simply Psychology*. https://www.simplypsychology.org/humanistic.html. Updated 2015.
10. John Brown, Sunbeams. *The Sun Magazine*, December 2014. http://thesunmagazine.org/issues/468/sunbeams.
11. Jack Kornfield, *A Lamp in the Darkness: Illuminating the Path Through Difficult Times*, Sounds True, Boulder, CO, 2011, p. 43.
12. UCLA Center for Mindfulness, About MARC. n.d. http://marc.ucla.edu/about-marc.
13. Atul Gawande, *Being Mortal: Medicine and What Matters in the End*, Metropolitan Books, Holt, New York, 2014, p. 188.
14. Schneider and Krug, *Existential–Humanistic Therapy*, p. 1.

CHAPTER 2 ▶ We're All in This Together

Individually, we are one drop. Together, we are an ocean.

—Ryunosuke Satoro[1]

Three Questions by Leo Tolstoy tells the story of a king who sought the answers to three important questions. It occurred to him that if he always knew the right time to begin everything; if he knew who were the right people to listen to, and whom to avoid; and, above all, if he always knew what was the most important thing to do, he would never fail in anything that he chose to do. So he had it proclaimed throughout his kingdom that he would give a great reward to anyone who would teach him what was the right time for every action, who were the most necessary people, and how he might know what was the most important thing to do.

The best minds and renowned experts from far and wide arrived at the castle, expounding learned theories and sage words, but none of their answers satisfied the king, who decided to set off on his own. Disguising himself in the clothes of a commoner, he set off to the hut of a wise hermit and arrived to find the man digging in his garden. The hermit was silent each time the king posed the questions, and as the day wore on, the king offered to dig for the hermit in order to give him some rest, all the while hoping that this might help his quest for knowledge. Time passed until a man emerged from the forest with a serious wound, which the king tended to, saving the man's life. After this long day, tired from his labors, the king slept in the hut of the hermit all that night. As morning came and the man was recovering from his wounds, he expressed gratitude to the king and told him that, in actuality, he had come to kill him to revenge the death of his brother and that, on his way, the king's guards had wounded him. All was forgiven by the man, who gave an oath of loyalty to the king and went on his way. The king then turned to the hermit and asked his three questions once again. The hermit responded that he, the king, had actually just had his questions answered. Because the king had stayed to help the exhausted hermit, he had avoided being killed by the man; by saving the man, he had allowed that man to forgive him; by taking care of the hermit and then the man, he was attending to who he was with in the present moment. The hermit advised the king of the following:

The most important time is now, the present is the only time over which we have power.
The most important person is the person you are with.
The most important thing is to do good to the person you are with.

This parable reminds us of the power of the present moment and the commitment to providing a healing environment in the work that we do with cancer survivors. It also speaks of taking the risk of being human with our patients rather than standing outside of ourselves, our patients, and our colleagues feeling disengaged, isolated, and lonely. This is an invitation to come home to the intentions that led us to the work we were called to do and a call to remember the heart of our work—human relationships. It is a chance to move from the paralyzing "us-versus-them" mentality that plagues cancer healthcare into a collaboration of patients, caregivers, and clinicians who feel appreciated, understood, and connected.

Providing quality emotional care for the growing number of cancer survivors has created an ongoing dilemma for all of us who are cancer healthcare professionals. Survivorship is a unique phase in overall cancer care, as people who are impacted by cancer may need support for years after their initial diagnosis and treatment. Chapter 1 introduced the history and background of the existential humanistic framework and suggested it as a good fit for working with this population. But how might we incorporate this perspective to enhance our clinical work, and what would it look like? How would it be applicable in the ongoing work with cancer survivors as well as for those who live with cancer? The questions of how to implement survivorship care can feel daunting; all too often we throw up our hands and give up hope that we can build quality survivorship programs that serve varied and diverse populations because the obstacles just seem too overwhelming. Providing services to help people with the emotional component of survivorship is both far-reaching and complex in nature, creating a need for collaboration among clinicians. The bigger picture of this reality requires an attention to implementing an accessible and doable approach to meet the needs of this growing population. For our purposes, introducing a simple, relational structure that allows both patients and clinicians to create a healing connection is one workable solution to the issues of quality survivorship care that can provide meaning and satisfaction to all concerned.

Cancer survivors are not one-size-fits-all, and their needs vary across a continuum, from those who have few long-term effects from their treatment to patients with chronic conditions or significant treatment-related health issues. Their relationships, their work lives, as well as their future plans have been forever altered. Nothing will ever be the same for them, and these realities are often overlooked when cancer patients feel rushed to move on and attain some illusion of a "new normal" without understanding and coming to terms with what they have been through. The good fortune of survival is clear, but the hidden disabilities and distresses that follow the patient, and their partners and families, can remain buried, leaving people silent in their suffering. The truth is, healing is a long haul, and the cancer healthcare system is struggling to assemble survivorship programs, resources, and referrals that will provide services for the emotional well-being of the growing number of survivors. It's daunting for providers to know what to do.

There are times when not knowing what to do *is* the truth, and you just have to stay with that until you do know what is needed and how to proceed. In today's world, we face numerous dilemmas in regard to caring for people in a difficult healthcare system. Inextricably interwoven with these dilemmas is the very serious predicament of caregiver burnout. As professionals committed to the work of healing, we have a mandate to do better both for our patients and for ourselves. During case consultation, my mentor, Dr. James Bugental, PhD, used to confront me when I muttered, "I don't know," while trying to understand a person or a situation; he said to me: "That's not good enough; you need to know." At this point in cancer survivorship care, it's not good enough to keep stalling out when we come face to face with the realities of finances, time, and energy. It's not good enough to end an exploration of possibilities by stating "That's just the way it is." As the wise wizard

Albus Dumbledore instructed Harry Potter: "Dark times lie ahead of us and there will be a time when we must choose between what is easy and what is right."[2]

Natasha Buchanan, PhD, behavioral scientist with the Epidemiology and Applied Research Branch of the Center for Disease Control and Prevention's Division of Cancer Prevention and Control, wrote:

The cancer experience may cause new psychosocial distress or exacerbate preexisting emotional, behavioral, and/or cognitive health concerns. Among those newly diagnosed with cancer and cancer survivors diagnosed with recurrent cancer, 20%–47% show a significant level of distress, and 17%– 75% of cancer survivors have reported concerns with memory, thinking, and attention, just after or several years after the end of treatment. The prevalence of psychosocial distress can vary by type of cancer, time since diagnosis, degree of physical impairment, amount of pain, prognosis, and other variables. Unfortunately, few cancer survivors (31%–37%) have had a discussion initiated by their doctors about psychosocial needs and concerns. And even fewer are receiving treatment for distress. Subsequently, less than half of distressed cancer survivors are actually identified and referred for psychosocial treatment and supportive services.[3]

A current definition of survivorship states that it begins at diagnosis. However, as a cancer survivor, my personal experience of survivorship did not begin at diagnosis. As a psychotherapist who works with cancer patients and their families, it is rare to hear of anyone who actually feels this way. The experience of feeling that you have survived cancer is unique to each individual, and, sadly, some people suffer from such extensive emotional trauma that they never quite believe that they will be well again and doubt that they have a future. It seems generally true that after the first year of post-treatment with clear scans, positive laboratory reports, and no evidence of disease, most people begin to draw a deeper breath and identify as a cancer survivor. However, the time it takes to shift an inner focus from cancer patient to cancer survivor cannot be, and should not be, generic, and no one should be judged or shamed for whatever time it takes to move through the trauma of a cancer diagnosis.

At the outset, the person diagnosed with cancer usually hits the ground running into treatment with little to no assurance that they will survive.

The time when the emotional consequences of all that has happened strikes unexpectedly, often after treatment ends or someone has been informed that their treatment will be ongoing. There are programs and groups for the newly diagnosed and those facing end-of-life concerns, but there is relatively little for those who survive cancer, so they are sent off on their own to fend for themselves.

Oncology providers are constantly pressed forward as their patient loads increase with each new wave of newly diagnosed patients appearing at the doorstep of their office. At the same time, their attention to those patients facing the end of life with terminal cancer, as well as their families, who are dealing with the impending loss, must also take precedence. Palliative care often has a clearer trajectory and, unfortunately, an imminent end, while those who are newly diagnosed are presented with various choices surrounding their treatment options, which is often a more pragmatic and concrete process. It feels impossible to manage the sheer number of people who need services.

As recognition of this growing group of survivors and the concerns of the providers who serve them become clear, the time to address the need for cancer survivor care that works for everyone is here. This calls on us to be mindful of the need for creativity, collaboration, and innovation when we focus on implementing survivorship care. We need to remember what brought us into cancer healthcare and what joins together in the work that we do.

Presence: Being Mindful of Ourselves and Others

Bringing ourselves into our work doesn't need to be that complicated. Being present with yourself and with the person you are with doesn't require that you have more work to do. You do not need to log a personal conversation into the database. Taking a moment to ask someone how they are conveys care and interest, and, perhaps even more significantly, it shows that you are curious about who that person is, that they are not just a patient or a number on a chart. There is potential for a level of simplicity in caring for your patients by allowing yourself to be present. There is always enough time when you are in the present moment.

The existential humanistic perspective focuses on people's innate drive for growth and the search for an authentic presence in life. This perspective applies to both the cancer patient and the cancer healthcare clinician. Patient- or person-centered care cannot work when it is one-sided; it needs to include both patient and provider to be balanced and effective. Building a healing relationship is at the heart of compassionate, meaningful person-centered cancer survivor care.

Jordan Grumet, an internal medicine physician and blogger (*In My Humble Opinion*) writes about assuring patients that we (doctors) are on their side in a blog on MedpageToday's KevinMD.com:

But there is something we can do to fight the colossal mess of what health care has become today. Instead of trying to explain the tangled mess of our lives to our patients, we should instead assure them that we are on their side. We should tell them that we won't stand for the destruction of humanism in medicine by the cold calculus of technology. We should tell them that we love them.[4]

These heartfelt words are a beautiful statement about the power of being present in a healing relationship. It also speaks to how being present as a clinician brings meaning into the work we do with our patients and our colleagues.

The practice of presence is different from the study of presence, or mindfulness as it is also sometimes currently known. It is experiential in nature and gained only by the commitment to work with being present both within yourself and with others. The ways to be present, to be mindful, can be learned by doing, and there are many accessible tools available. But to become more authentically present requires times of introspection and a developed capacity to honor another human being for who the person is and where he or she is in life. To become more present with others demands attention to bringing empathy, honesty, clear communication, and intimacy into your relationships. Discovering what keeps you from being as fully present as you can be with others is the best way to shift habitual and deadening patterns in relationships.

When I can truly "be with"—and I am not saying this happens all the time or even often in any kind of predictable way—I can find peace and a restorative energy. So my level of need becomes a function of how much

I am resisting the sometimes intractable difficulties of my clients, how hard I am working to fix unfixable things, how distressed I am by the parameters of human life.

—Merideth Shamszad, Psychotherapist, email interview, July 3, 2016

Presence is a learned skill and an ongoing practice. But what does it mean to be present, and how do we continue to stay in the present moment with all the demands and requirements of our work? People assume that you are either present or not present, often ascribing mystical powers to the concept only found in monks living in Himalayan caves. However, learning to be present is possible, is not static, and is, by its nature, continually changing without an end point. Over time, it becomes a way of being in the world and can be instrumental in finding and maintaining a personal and professional balance in your life that is fluid and satisfactory.

James Bugental wrote that "*Presence* is a name for the quality of being in a situation or relationship in which one intends at a deep level to participate as fully as she is able."[5] In further chapters as we move into the pragmatic application of this definition, we'll look at the differences between taking charge and the illusion of being in control, how personal boundaries affect the life–work balance, being in touch with your intuitive mind, trusting change and uncertainty in difficult situations and with difficult people, and, finally, the freedom of letting go into the present moment. The workbook sections of this book provide tools and resources you can lean on to help you develop ways of being present and mindful in your work and, of course, your life.

Moving from Illness to Wellness

The first year following treatment is a key time in the emotional recovery from a cancer diagnosis. One of my clients, a young breast cancer patient who had endured a complicated medical history since childhood, walked into my office essentially feeling hopeless that she would remain cancer-free. Her life experience had taught her that she couldn't trust her body to be strong and healthy; truthfully, she had a great deal of personal experience to back up these fears. Her distress and anxiety had been pathologized by numerous providers, leaving her feeling alone and ashamed. When her experience was validated as real and she was allowed her thoughts and feelings, she began to bring herself into the present moment, a moment where she could experience that she was growing healthy after treatment. In the months that followed, she gained a new trust in herself, in her body, and began to believe not only that she would live, but also that she would grow, take risks, and enjoy her life. She had accessed her innate drive for wellness and growth and left my office stating, "I'm more interested in living my life and having new experiences than being in therapy." Given the chance to tell her story, she found her way through the dark tunnel of her fears of recurrence and into the light of living her life as fully as possible in the present moment each day.

We need to create a safe space to hear our client's story.

—Dolores Moorehead, Patient Care Navigator, oral interview, July 22, 2016

As clinicians, we must understand that follow-up care needs to be dynamic and that the goals or intentions of the care plan must be fluid to consistently assess and address the changing needs of the survivor. Survivorship care differs from palliative care in that the attention is on moving forward into wellness, processing how one has been affected by cancer, and exploring how one will make choices affecting one's future. The nature of this existential searching is not a short-term process and therefore becomes important to present as a long-term venture that moves beyond brief behavioral modalities that are effective for different circumstances.

The need for follow-up cancer care that addresses physical well-being is more obvious and concrete than is the psychological component of survivorship, which can touch the areas of personal and emotional concerns that are related to physical issues and trauma. Helping survivors assimilate their experience matters as it is now well acknowledged that the mind, body, soul connection is a valid perspective in integrated healthcare. It is important to note that survivors are members of a complex network of individuals, including family members and caregivers; all members of the network experience stresses from the cancer diagnosis, including depression, job security or work issues, and financial strains, which may vary across time. The entire group is moving from a period of illness and cancer treatment into healing and wellness. Giving attention to the vulnerable landscape of entering wellness after an illness fosters an aliveness and curiosity to cancer survivors' transition from the treatment room to the new rooms of their lives in the days, months, and years following their cancer experience. If the perspective of personal growth is offered during this phase of survivorship along with the resources to support a reflective exploration, the possibilities of a deep and meaningful healing experience are greatly expanded. By presenting people with the personal responsibility not only for their own recovery but also for the opportunity to transform their experience, we give them the gift of trust in their capacity to move forward in meaningful ways.

The will to live cannot be measured, which puts it beyond the reach of science. Science defines life in its own ways but often life is larger than science. People are larger than science, too. Many important things cannot be measured or even predicted but only experienced. So the Medicine of the future needs to be larger than its science as well.

—Rachel Naomi Remen, MD, "The Power of Wholeness"[6]

This humanistic stance enhances the possibility of streamlining your assessment of your patient, as you often learn more about them from the contact you have with them than from the usual distress screening forms. This could also be the juncture where you gain knowledge and insight into their emotional state so that you can help them determine their psychosocial needs and offer appropriate referrals. Basic skills in communication require very little time and energy to learn and will enhance the quality of your interactions with patients, which in the end will mutually benefit all. Honoring your own humanity creates a trusting atmosphere that allows you and those you are in relationship with to relax and open up. This acknowledgment of the imperfect and uncertain circumstances in which we work and live ironically facilitates the lessening of fearfulness and being overwhelmed. In his book *The Laws of Medicine*, Siddhartha Mukherjee writes about what he learned from his experience as a medical student: "Looking back, I realize that I lived for a year, perhaps two, like a clockwork human, moving from one subroutine to the next. Days folded into identical days, all set to the same rhythm. By the end of my first month, even 'flex' had turned into reflex."[7] As I read more and more pieces written by medical students who endure depression and despair and acquaint myself with the distress that students and physicians experience, I am even more convinced of the importance of humanizing healthcare for all concerned.

Along with naming the issues faced by cancer providers, it is equally valuable for clinicians who are working with cancer survivors to educate themselves in regard to the themes that are prevalent in cancer survivorship:

- Living with uncertainty
- Issues of mortality
- Identity struggles after cancer
- Body image issues
- Loss
- Quality of life
- Anxiety
- Depression
- Self-criticism over emotional responses

This doesn't mean that you need to be an expert in all the complexities of a cancer diagnosis, but it does mean that you educate yourself enough to know where to go to cultivate an understanding of the particular issues that cancer survivors face. There can be a common misunderstanding that everyone faces these issues. Things like uncertainty, for instance, are universal. While that is true, it is not true that these concerns are the same for those who have been impacted by a life-threatening illness. Having an understanding of these specific issues prevents a misunderstanding, and misdiagnosis, of anxiety and depression as a pathological problem rather than knowing it as part of the emotional landscape. Judging the anxieties, depression, and fears that are common for cancer survivors only creates an atmosphere of shame, which leads to survivors becoming self-critical and unable to express the trauma they have been through.

It isn't just the theory behind the problems that shows up in numbers, statistics and spreadsheets; health care is a complex beast that requires detailed understanding and knowledge of the frontline clinical processes and systems. In this arena, there's no substitute for experience, common sense, and understanding people. Health care isn't like buying a sofa or visiting a restaurant or hotel. Experience, sincerity and being able to put yourself in your patients' shoes will produce the real leaders of the future. We need fewer doctor MBAs and more trusted doctor healers.

—Suneel Dhand, MD, "We Need Fewer Doctor MBAs and More Doctor Healers"[8]

Truthfully, most patients don't expect their physicians or healthcare providers to spend a great deal of time with them. No one is naïve to the limitations that providers face in their daily practice. However, a kind word, a brief check in, an apology for a long wait—all mean a great deal. Our path toward collaborative survivorship care is to see through the patient's eyes, acknowledge their experience, and help them reflect on their journey. Alongside this care for our patients, we must also acknowledge our own experience and spend time personally reflecting on our own lives. When we allow ourselves to be compassionate with ourselves and with others in our work, a world of meaningful opportunities to do better opens up to us.

Referral and Resources: Helping One Another Out

Most agencies are grateful that another person is on the team. When we connect around a case and someone knows that we are here to help, I can hear an audible exhale on the other end of the phone.

—Cassandra Falby, MFT, Program Director, Women's Cancer Resource Center

Cancer survivors need a certain amount of independence and self-advocacy skills in order to effectively navigate the healthcare system and find services for themselves and their families. Cultural, socioeconomic, and logistical issues all affect the ability to advocate for oneself, and not everyone has the capacity to handle some of the barriers to their care. Cancer clinicians may not have the time or space to provide care for survivors dealing with the long-term or late effects of cancer due to their high numbers in their patient load. We need to confront the barriers to communication between the different treatment teams; these barriers seem to be based in the fear of referring to other clinicians and a lack of willingness to identify the emotional factors in cancer survivorship as a valid issue. These disparities in providing quality emotional care occur largely due to lack of communication skills training for health-care providers, a competitive attitude learned by necessity in high-pressure education and training, and a misunderstanding of the value of attending to the mind–body connection in healing from the trauma of cancer that leads to a lack of referral to experienced psychotherapeutic professionals.

It is possible to put together available resources for survivors rather than staying stuck on the difficulties involving lack of resources. This requires openness to using existing resources with the help of a competent navigation network of providers that includes oncologists, radiologists, nurses, social workers, psychotherapists, and practitioners of complimentary medicine (e.g., acupuncture), who are all open and willing to collaborate with one another. There are often concerns of losing patients to other practitioners, but what is important to remember is that there are different clinicians who are experienced and prepared to work with the complex issues of survivorship. Clinical scope of practice requires that we work within the boundaries of our education, professional experience, and what we are licensed to offer. Veering too far off course from that scope is both ineffective and dangerous. Professional collaboration between these disciplines forms a network of providers that better serves the patients and has the potential of forming strong collegial bonds between clinicians.

Bringing theory into practice requires building alliances not only with patients but also with other professionals. This necessitates a joint venture between the medical team, social workers, clinics, and psychotherapists. Each group has its expertise—when the need is medical, refer to the medical team; when the need is psychological, refer to the psychotherapist; when the need is psychosocial, refer to the social worker. Coordinating resources and making appropriate referrals is a major key to creating successful survivorship care. There is a powerful web of providers, and together we can actualize a humanistic system that benefits both our patients and ourselves.

Most places have someone called a navigator but the definition of the reality varies significantly. The burden is on the patient to coordinate their care, for the most part. The referring doctor's office rarely takes responsibility for making sure the patient gets that appointment, knows where to go and what to expect and what questions the patient may have after the visit. That is the minimum that I consider true navigation.

—Meridithe Mendelsohn, Program Manager, Cancer Survivorship, email interview, July 18, 2016

The bare minimum of effective navigation involves concrete tasks, such as referrals, appointments, and scheduled follow-ups, and this does not even begin to touch a level of quality care for patients. To improve communication and coordination among providers and patients and between different providers, discussions about the post-treatment transition should begin before survivors end their treatment. Giving survivors, family members, and caregivers education on resources, as well as appropriate referrals to needed services, will aid them in their own self-advocacy and create a network between clinicians that can build a foundation for quality survivorship care.

An Authentic Survivorship Plan

We need to create education and training programs and accessible resource materials to help clinicians learn communication skills and find ways to connect with one another. This text provides workbook space for this purpose, and there can be a great advantage to using the already available technological tools that help clinicians share information as well as connect with one another. Regular texts and brief email contact between clinicians can be structured so they do not violate confidentiality for the patients and, perhaps even more helpfully, can be a way for clinicians to check in and support one another during stressful times.

Here's what we can do:

- Create patient-centered survivorship care
- Create a humanistic system for cancer healthcare providers
- Develop educational programs on awareness of cancer survivorship issues
- Include psychological support to complement medically focused oncology care

- Develop a directory of community resources and referral options for survivors and providers
- Help individuals navigate and access the healthcare system
- Develop outreach programs, resources, and guidance to assist community providers to provide long-term care for cancer survivors
- Create online services and satellite clinics to service remote areas
- Implement specialized teams of both medical and psychosocial clinicians at cancer centers, clinics, private practice settings

Survivors need to know that they have a place to come after they have finished treatment. In many ways, it really doesn't matter where this is or even what this is, just that it exists. It's important for them to be able to communicate their thoughts and feelings as that offers a sense of belonging that fosters healing. As clinicians, we are committed to serving this population, and this requires that we help build a structure for quality survivorship care piece by piece with one another.

Alone we cannot change what is broken; together we have a chance to make a difference. There is enough suffering in the cancer healthcare system that we cannot change; we must turn our attention to what can be transformed so that both patient and provider are served in meaningful ways. This is not about just one person—the change we want to see in our work requires partnership and collaboration between all of us. This is not a monologue or a solo performance, it requires that people who care band together, find our voices, and speak out loud.

The following narrative questions are designed to help you focus on your questions and concerns as a clinician working with cancer survivors. Becoming aware and mindful is not some esoteric cure. Awareness is the important first part of change, but it also requires action to be effective. Your problems will not automatically disappear without both your insight regarding transformation and your commitment to participating in the changes you want to see. To be mindful and awake is not some magical state without any problems. Finding the courage to acknowledge the way things are, to assess what can be changed, to trust the present moment to guide you where you need to be, allows your humanness to serve as a foundation for meaningful work with cancer survivors. Supporting yourself and other healthcare practitioners in their professional lives, addressing the vital issue of work–life balance, restoring a sense of personal meaning, and understanding what quality of life means to you, are all essential steps to moving forward in the creation of a humanistic cancer care system.

1. What is your work? How is it going these days?

   _____

   _____

   _____

   _____

2. What are your concerns about providing quality survivorship care to your patients/clients? Ask yourself, Are my patients getting what I want them to have from me?

   _____

   _____

   _____

   _____

3. What would help you provide this care? Ask yourself, Am I getting what I need in order to do my work?

_____

_____

_____

_____

4. What do you see as the barriers to implementing quality survivorship care?

_____

_____

_____

_____

5. What do you see as possible solutions to these barriers?

_____

_____

_____

_____

6. Describe a model of cancer survivorship care that integrates the emotional component of healing from a cancer diagnosis.

_____

_____

_____

_____

7. At the end of the day . . . how would you like to feel in your work?

_____

_____

_____

_____

8. Reflect on how you would like to humanize your work with your patients/clients. Allow yourself to imagine how you want this to look and feel.

_____

_____

_____

_____

9. What do you do not to lose your humanity?

_____

_____

_____

_____

Notes

1. Ryunosuke Satoro, Ryunosuke Satoro Quotes, BrainyQuote. 2017. https://www.brainyquote.com/quotes/quotes/r/ryunosukes167565.html. Accessed April 18, 2017.

2. J. K. Rowling, *Harry Potter and the Goblet of Fire*. Bloomsbury, England: Scholastic, US. July 8, 2000. https://www.goodreads.com/quotes/701025-dark-times-lie-ahead-of-us-and-there-will-be

3. Natasha Buchanan, PhD, Alleviate Cancer Survivor Distress: Screening and Psychosocial Care. http://www.medscape.com/viewarticle/864507. Published June 20, 2016.

4. Jordan Grumet, MD, Assure Patients That We Are on Their Side. KevinMD.com. http://www.kevinmd.com/blog/2014/03/assure-patients-side.html. Published March 28, 2014.

5. James F. T. Bugental, *The Art of the Psychotherapist*, Norton, New York, 1987, p. 27.

6. Rachel Naomi Remen, MD, The Power of Wholeness. http://www.rachelremen.com/the-power-of-wholeness/. Published January 11, 2013.

7. Siddhartha Mukherjee MD, *The Laws of Medicine: Field Notes from an Uncertain Science*, Ted Books, Simon and Schuster, New York, 2015, p. 11.

8. Suneel Dhand, MD, We Need Fewer Doctor MBAs and More Doctor Healers. KevinMD.com. http://www.kevinmd.com/blog/2014/06/need-fewer-doctor-mbas-doctor-healers.html. Published June 20, 2014.

CHAPTER 3

The Healing Power of Authenticity

Person-Centered Communication in Survivorship Care

> *I was taught to always offer a gown,*
> *frequently folded inside out,*
> *and tell the patient, Put the opening*
> *behind and this sheet across your lap.*
> *In the next step, I learned to uncover*
> *the roots of bewilderment, beginning*
> *with the eyes and continuing down,*
>
> *a performance laden with gesture,*
> *encouraging hope, I delivered my script.*
> *And you, my intimate companion,*
> *you were consigned to endure the suspense*
> *of me reading a narrative in your flesh.*

—Jack Coulehan, MD, "Take Off Your Clothes"[1]

Because listening can bring about such powerful healing, it is one of the most beautiful gifts that people can give and receive.

—Carl Faber, PhD, *On Listening*[2]

All authentic communication begins with listening. Being seen, heard, and understood for who you are and where you are in the given moments of your life involve a basic human need that is as important as being able to take your next breath. This essential aspect of relationship is the bedrock of effective communication and actually does not mean long, drawn-out conversations and wordy interactions as much as it means offering a personal stance of respect and care felt and conveyed by both clinician and patient. In many ways, the type of treatment plan a patient chooses to follow doesn't matter as much as an authentic connection to the practitioner, which gives the patient respect, recognition, and the chance to be fully present. Meeting someone directly takes no more time than relating from a place of disengagement and, the killer of truly effective communication, objectivity. The act of authentic listening becomes a place to gather for connection, growth, and healing.

It's more than likely that you feel the impact of "cost-effective" measures that are eroding the real work of healing. Atul Gawande, MD, in a piece in the August 2012 *New Yorker* magazine, "Big Med," compared the business of medicine with the business model of the Cheesecake Factory. He wrote:

Our new models come from industries that have learned to increase the capabilities and efficiency of human beings who work for them. Yet the same industries have also tended to devalue those employees. The frontline worker, whether he is making cars, solar panels, or wasabi-crusted ahi tuna, now generates unprecedented value but receives little of the wealth he is creating. Can we avoid this as we revolutionize healthcare?[3]

Gawande goes on to talk about what he perceives as an inevitable switch to "health care chains" that will impact the providers working within them. He makes a strong statement about nurses and doctors working in a healthcare system where their "convenience" will come second to the patient's "experience." No longer feeling connected with the work of healing, you find yourself drowning in a sea of paperwork and unfulfilling tasks.

The challenge, therefore, is to remain human in a robotic system where the temptation to retreat into a depersonalized position is enormous. Too often, your patient interactions are swift and impersonal, like going through the drive-through at a fast food chain. I believe this is what's at the heart of the loss of meaning and inspiration for most care providers. When you feel trapped in the role of technician, you lose the connection with both your patients and yourself. The frayed threads of inner connection will leave you feeling lost and lonely. Meaningful work fades into rote tasks performed *on* others rather than being a relational process *between* patient/client and provider. When you add this to feeling like a cog in the wheel of a factory delivery system, you will have a depressing, debilitating work life.

There are ways to deal with the demanding work that you do. You may be surprised to discover that it only takes a few moments to check in with the emotional concerns of your patients, and that in doing so you can add to the quality of your relationship with that person. Listening deeply to your patient is a way to get to know them and helps guide you in accurate assessments; it also helps you to make the necessary referrals for psychotherapy or other integrative practices. In this chapter, we look at ways to incorporate the existential humanistic perspective into primary communication skills for use in the work you do with cancer survivors.

In an email interview on July 20, 2016, with Dr. Jon Greif, retired oncology breast surgeon and research investigator (National Institute of Health, NIH), I asked what he believed to be helpful (and not helpful) for providers of cancer care. He wrote the following:

Healthcare providers need to know what their patients regard as important, and not important, and even detrimental to their cancer care experience—reporting the experience from the patient's and her/his family and support network's perspective would be most helpful. A rehash of the usual provider complaints (not enough time, too much "paper work," inadequate compensation, lack of administrative support, etc.) would not be helpful.

Survivors are sometimes given instructions for how they are supposed to talk to their providers, things like what to ask and when to listen. They're constantly being told to advocate for themselves (the companion to this text, *Surviving the Storm* [Krauter, 2017], discusses this). By the same measure, clinicians must communicate clearly and listen to and advocate not only for their patients but also for themselves. Relationships by their very nature are two-sided, and it takes both people being willing to reach out a hand to another human being. During the writing of this book, I spoke with Dolores Moorehead, Patient Care Navigator, who put it beautifully when she said, "The clinician needs to be in a space of support and encouragement. Being real has a heart to heart connection."

The goal of this chapter is to enhance the quality of communication between patient and provider. It presents exercises and examples of skillful communication techniques that can be adapted by clinicians for needs assessment, emotional evaluation, distress screening, and satisfying interactions in cancer healthcare while also taking into account the individual style, boundaries, and personal choices made by each individual clinician. You are invited to explore the questions, exercises, and skills in the workbook section at the end of this chapter.

You can go on by doing the best you can. You can go on by being generous. You can go on by being true. You can go on by offering comfort to others who can't go on. You can go on by allowing the unbearable days to pass and by allowing the pleasure in other days. You can go on by finding a channel for your love and another for your rage.

—Cheryl Strayed, *Brave Enough*[4]

Bringing an Open Heart to Work

In our work with cancer survivors, we are continually faced with very real human concerns circling around life and death. We are called to sit with people who face tremendous fear, confusion, and pain as they traverse the trials of cancer survivorship. Their stories spring out of the reality of their experience as a human being who is confronting a life-threatening illness, which by its very nature of threatening a person's existence can bring about an existential crisis. In *The Art of the Psychotherapist,* James Bugental, PhD, wrote:

The basic theory of this psychotherapy is called existential because it has to do with the fact of existence. The value orientation of this psychotherapy is called humanistic because it sees the greater realization of the potentials of human beings as the most desirable outcome of the therapeutic work. Existential anxiety, the anxiety of being, is anxiety that cannot be analyzed away.[5]

An existential confrontation of the soul cannot be fit into a prescribed or generic program that only attends to behavioral changes and offers ways to adapt to a situation rather than pursue the avenue of awareness and transformation. Bringing the basic tenants of an existential humanistic perspective into the interactions with survivors is in alignment with their very real experiences and helps them to move through their recovery and healing in a meaningful way. By bringing the humanistic perspective to their part of this existential searching, the clinician joins with their patient in the experience of what it means to be human. And let's not overlook the fact that working in cancer healthcare also puts you, as a clinician, in an ongoing stream of existential moments both with others and within yourself.

Survivors who confront the existential crisis of life-threatening illness take time to reflect, and from that place of reflection they make choices that impact them in positive ways, often emerging more creative and grateful in their lives. These people invariably report that it was the awareness of having the support and care of their provider that was the most valuable part of their treatment. It's comforting and sustaining merely to know that they mattered to those who were treating them. When the clinician lets the patient matter to him or her and then meets the existential dilemmas of being alive while struggling with illness and healing with a willingness to engage at a personal level, the clinician brings an aliveness into his or her work with survivors. Bringing your love into your work is a way to keep your heart open.

The First Year After Treatment

The most effective time to begin addressing the issues of survivorship occurs just prior to finishing treatment. At this point, the survivor is starting to look ahead to what's next for them, as well as dealing with the thoughts and feelings of ending their cancer treatment. This is a key time for successful interventions that involve helping the survivor with both the physical and emotional trauma of a cancer diagnosis. It's important to include the partners, family members, and caregivers in this conversation as they have also survived their own storm. Starting these conversations before the patient moves into the post-treatment phase helps to set up a structure or plan for them to use and rely on as they head into the uncertain territory of survivorship.

Attending to the needs of your patients will differ depending on your specific clinical role and the services you provide. If you are an oncologist, your contact will likely be a brief check-in rather than a longer session, as might be the case with a psychotherapist. But no matter what your role is, this work is not about "fixing" someone, but rather about bringing authentic communication into whatever type of work you do. It's important to remember that you cannot take responsibility for someone else's choices or actions. You are not responsible for someone else's life. When you can fully accept this reality, you will free yourself to listen more deeply and let go of the attachment to your patient's life choices being your responsibility. Ironically, letting go of feeling overresponsible for another person frees you to be more fully responsible for the real commitment of care, which is to hold your patient with love and respect in the service of their healing. Our responsibility as clinicians is to support the growth of our patients and to contribute both our knowledge and our care on behalf of their well-being.

In all the cancer-related talks, workshops, and events I have attended, as well as those where I've presented, I have found a great need for survivors to speak about their experiences. They want to tell their stories. When they have the opportunity to tell the entirety of what they've gone through—starting at the end of their treatment and into the first year of survivorship—they tend to release trauma rather than carry it inside as long or as deeply.

There is certainly value for survivors in telling their story at any point in their healing, but the recovery is smoother and happens sooner when they are given the chance to speak about what has happened for them. This experience offers the patient an opportunity to feel met and that their practitioner is listening. And you gain valuable insight into both their physical and their emotional states by hearing what they have to say. Through the simple act of telling, of being witnessed while they paint the pictures of their experience, they find a certain relief, a freedom in releasing what has been held and carried. Speaking the trauma liberates the patient from what could be days, months, and even years of distress due to an unprocessed emotional experience. Let's look at how you can help your patients tell their stories at the beginning of survivorship so that they may begin the process of healing sooner rather than later.

The Four *C*'s of Communication

- **Communication** begins with making contact by simply asking someone, "How are you?" The next step is to be as fully present as possible as you listen to what they have to say. As obvious as this may seem, "to be genuinely present is no small matter."[6] Create a safe space for people to feel that they have an open avenue of communication that includes a structure for feedback from patients, their partners, and their families.

- **Curiosity** about the person sitting in front of you. Being engaged and involved in the interactions that you have with your patients conveys to them that you are interested in who they are as another human being, not just a number on a chart.

- **Concern** is the internal experience of discovering and valuing what matters to you in the service of taking yourself and your life seriously. You have to care enough about yourself to make difficult choices and then dig deep to make the changes that are important to your well-being. "Concern is a name for the attitude and emotional set of a person who seriously considers his own life and the course it is taking."[7] Finding concern includes not only helping your patients but also paying attention to what concerns you both professionally and personally.

- **Conversation** is a parallel process of dialogue between people with the intention of clarity. In essence, it is our responsibility as clinicians to be sure that we are on the same page, particularly during important conversations. We must be aware of whether or not our patient understands what we are saying and use language that is easily understood. This entails paying attention to the verbal and, especially, nonverbal cues of the patient and incorporating ways to check in with the person throughout the conversation to avoid misunderstanding and incorrect assumptions.

The Importance of Recognizing and Understanding Universal Cancer Survivor Themes

Cancer changes people, yes, but what exactly has been altered isn't clear at the moment someone receives a diagnosis. It's not possible to know how your life will change before you have the experience of living it. Authentic transformation shows itself over time when we pay attention, give attention, and allow awareness to emerge. And while every person has a unique cancer experience, there are certain themes that appear common to those who have drawn the short straw of cancer. It's useful to clinicians to be aware of these concerns as valid and not to deny their existence. Clinicians need to educate themselves to the signs and signals of emotional distress, learn how to recognize normal responses to trauma, and pay close attention to what patients mark on their distress screening form. Recognition and understanding of these emotional concerns leads to effective psychosocial referrals from medical professionals. People who have been traumatized by cancer deserve our patience and our empathy. In an email interview on July 2, 2016, Merideth Shamszad, MFT, put it beautifully in this comment: "We need to be able to sit in our sometimes massive, raw fear (our own or our clients'), our mammalian selves, our cultures, without heading for the nearest 'fixit' escape. If we do that we can sometimes encounter with our clients that place I call 'grace', marked by an ease and a surrender that are awe-inspiring."

The following themes are addressed in the workbook section following this chapter.

- Living with uncertainty
- Issues of mortality
- Identity struggles after cancer
- Body image issues
- Loss
- Quality of life
- Anxiety
- Depression
- Self-criticism over emotional responses

Coming from an existential perspective of looking at cancer survivorship means that we are not looking at the classic story structure of beginning, middle, and end but are instead working with a more circular framework of experience. This is why I advocate for utilizing a narrative interview as a more effective method for both survivors and clinicians. Open-ended questions will yield far more accurate and extensive personal information about the patient, which then supports the clinician's skillful assessment. This narrative structure in and of itself opens up the human quality of the interview, which is productive for both the patient and the clinician in the aliveness of its contact. The medical setting has become so big and unwieldy that the patient can get lost in computer records, paperwork, backlogged appointments, and unreturned phone calls. They feel like a number because, in truth, they *have* become a number in the mass of the numbers of patients. In a variation of that theme, this very same system has seriously affected the dehumanizing experience of clinicians. This loss of authentic connection for both patient and clinician is at the root of despair in the healthcare community. According to James Bugental[8]:

By authenticity I mean a genuineness and awareness of being. Authenticity is that presence of an individual in his living in which he is fully aware in the present moment in the present situation. Authenticity is difficult to convey in words, but experientially it is readily perceived in ourselves or in others.

There are ways to encourage and integrate authenticity even within the limitations of the current medical system. The most essential aspects of this are first to acknowledge that disconnected and inauthentic communication is a problem, and second to know that it can be resolved. Our work will not be perfect, and it will not always go the way we want it to. What we provide only needs to be good enough for people to realize that they do not have to continue in a disenfranchised and depressing system. This involves education in communication skills for clinicians beginning in medical school and extending throughout their careers, a commitment to personal awareness, and knowing when to refer to psychosocial professionals.

In my book *Surviving the Storm: A Workbook for Telling Your Cancer Story* (2017), I offer a series of open-ended questions that provide a good place to start. Practitioners can recommend this workbook to their patients as they begin their journey into survivorship.

A Time to Talk
When a friend calls to me from the road
And slows his horse to a meaning walk,
I don't stand still and look around
On all the hills I haven't hoed,
And shout from where I am, What is it?
No, not as there is a time to talk.
I thrust my hoe in the mellow ground,
Blade-end up and five feet tall,
And plod: I go up to the stone wall
For a friendly visit.

—Robert Frost, from "Mountain Interval"[9]

Human authenticity is to be searching, realizing, moving on, searching, arriving, and moving on again.

—James Bugental, *The Search for Authenticity*[10]

Bringing a humanistic touch to the care of others means that our interactions are not based on techniques or tools but rather a personal and relational awareness that, in and of itself, creates a genuine connection in the healing relationship. While science and medicine are evidence-based in nature, a skillful, personal interview is more of an art than a scientific study. A thoughtful clinician develops himself or herself in much the same as any artist perfects his or her craft, combining talent, skill, and hard work that is honed through education, practice, feedback, and a commitment to the artistry of authentic connection. Helping our patients to move into survivorship in a way that creates genuine healing requires that we work together to create an individualized plan for each person. The success of these plans depends on educating our patients, providing appropriate referrals, and helping them to learn how they can identify and negotiate their needs for themselves as they move forward.

As clinicians, there is an art to guiding people through the stormy waters of cancer survivorship that includes compassion, good communication, and a strong professional stance while also being open and willing to go outside the prescribed boxes provided on the standard and generic screening forms used in cancer healthcare. The art of the interview often means that we color outside of the lines by being willing to give more attention to the person we are with, rather than relying on a set of diagnostic tools or rigid rules that objectify our patients. Each relationship is unique, and it is important to acknowledge and allow this subjectivity to inform how we work with people as individuals.

There is a current conversation about returning to more "old school" practices of medicine that include touch, listening, and taking time with patients; these fall under the category of "the art of medicine." This conversation opens up a controversial topic when it's applied to actual medical procedures as clinicians sometimes feel concerned that evidence-based scientific measures will fall by the wayside in clinical work. At the heart of the healing relationship is another kind of art—the "art of the interaction," which focuses on the quality of communication between clinician and patient. This book introduces a person-centered approach rather than just a patient-centered approach to include the clinician as an important part of the interaction. This is vitally important, as the essence of person-centered care is an authentic connection between clinician and patient because it moves away from the imbalance of power that often occurs in clinical relationships. This framework demands that both individuals be present and responsive in the interaction with an intention of awareness and understanding. Indeed, rather than adding to your workload, this more connected and authentic communication is actually a preventive measure for burnout because you're part of a meaningful process (Chapter 6 discusses self-care). Genuine contact and care call for the conscious participation of the clinician, are not based on techniques or "canned lines and responses," and fundamentally rest on your personal qualities as the basis of an empathic relationship. For this to work well, it requires that you bring developed personal awareness and commitment to consciousness to your work.

The Authentic Clinician: Ourselves

Nobody wants to be told on an answering machine or in an email that they have cancer. In our line of work, we need a more personal approach all the way through the process, which continues during the transition from cancer patient to cancer survivor. The balance of recovering from medical treatment and the emotional healing from cancer includes evidence-based perspectives woven together with the importance of a human viewpoint that builds a subjective framework for the physical and emotional needs of cancer survivors.

Subjectivity is that inner, separate, and private realm in which we live most genuinely. The simple but profound truth, is that we are subjects rather than objects, actors not the acted-upon, and this sovereignty is the essence of our subjectivity. Therein lies the ultimate meaning: It is the autonomy of human beings which escapes the cages of objective determinism and which resides in our subjectivity.

—James F. T. Bugental, *The Art of the Psychotherapist*[11]

Learning how to be skillful in our contact with others is the art of a therapeutic interaction and is something that can be learned and developed. Like any art, it needs continued attention and practice and involves a commitment to broadening and deepening our capacity to authentically relate to another human being. Moving away from an objective viewpoint of treating another human being, we rely on our subjective experience, our sensitivity, and our empathy. We need to be with people, not "work on" them as if they were a car or a microwave. The most compelling aspect of the art of a healing interaction is the ability to be present within ourselves and meet the person we are with where they are in their own experience. By developing our own intuition, self-awareness, and understanding of others, we bring our best selves into a healing relationship. When our hearts are open, we communicate with a sense of abundance and expansiveness, which allows us to be human with ourselves and, therefore, with others. We are free to connect with the person we are sitting with where they are in the present moment.

The Clinician's Use of Self

Being present and caring are what make up the fundamental ground for healing. Being present is first an "inside job," meaning that you always start by being present within yourself to be present with others. The questions that follow can help you explore and find ways to listen to your inner voice in order to be present, alert, involved, and genuinely emotionally resonant in your daily life. You can be your best support system and have your own back by learning to tune in to your own inner world.

Being Present

1. How do I pay attention to myself?

_____

_____

_____

_____

2. Do I create time and space for myself to reflect on myself and my work?

_____

_____

_____

_____

3. If you answered no to the last question, how might you create time and space for yourself? Think about places, times, active or passive moments that you recognize as ways you can feel in touch with yourself.

_____

_____

_____

_____

4. Do you feel like you pay attention to yourself on a regular basis? How do you do this? If this feels distant to you, what might help remind you to check in with yourself?

_____

_____

_____

_____

5. Is it okay to pay attention to yourself during a busy or stressful workday? How do you tune in to yourself when the demands of your work are high?

_____

_____

6. Do you have any kind of practice that helps you focus on yourself, that helps you learn how to be present? If so, what is this practice?

_____

_____

_____

_____

7. Would you like to learn how to give better attention to yourself? What do you imagine that this would look like, feel like, and be like for you? Think about or visualize this for yourself and see what you discover.

_____

_____

_____

_____

Being with the Challenges of Work

1. What are some of the current challenges of your work?

_____

_____

_____

_____

2. Are some of these challenges ongoing? How is this for you?

_____

_____

_____

_____

3. Do you experience your work as an evolving process with room for growth?

_____

_____

_____

_____

4. Do you sometimes fight against feelings of resignation when the challenges of your work feel too daunting?

_____

_____

_____

_____

5. What helps you understand how the challenges of your work affect you? Do you allow yourself to pay attention to how these issues impact you?

_____

_____

_____

_____

6. What concerns you about your work? Allow yourself to write what arises, freely and without hesitation. Let yourself trust what comes up.

_____

_____

_____

_____

Developing a Disciplined Sensitivity

1. Are you in touch with your own intuition? If so, how do you recognize this part of yourself?

_____

_____

_____

_____

2. How do you access your intuition? Is this aspect of consciousness available to you?

_____

_____

_____

_____

3. Do you use your intuition in your work? Is intuition a personal tool that enhances your senses and receptivity to yourself and others?

_____

_____

_____

_____

4. Are you comfortable with different states and intensities of emotion within yourself? What helps you to be accepting of different emotional states?

_____

_____

_____

_____

5. Are you comfortable with sensitive subjects or moments with your patients/clients? What happens inside of you during these times?

_____

_____

_____

_____

6. What's your experience of your own sensitivity as a clinician? Do you believe it to be an asset or a liability?

_____

_____

_____

_____

7. Are you concerned that if you come from a place of sensitivity you will be overwhelmed or seen as "weak or incompetent" by your colleagues?

_____

_____

_____

_____

8. How do you see the connection between sensitivity and empathy?

_____

_____

_____

_____

9. What value do you see in cultivating your sensitivity as a way to enliven the work that you do?

_____

_____

_____

_____

Continuing to Grow and Develop

1. What kind of activity or study do you engage in for your professional growth and development?

    _____

    _____

    _____

    _____

2. What courses would you find stimulating and relevant to your professional growth and development?

    _____

    _____

    _____

    _____

3. Would you find a retreat an experience that would rejuvenate you as well as provide moments of rest and relaxation?

    _____

    _____

    _____

    _____

4. What value do you see in an ongoing commitment to your professional development that integrates your physical, emotional, mental growth with your professional competency?

    _____

    _____

    _____

    _____

5. Do you bring a curious and self-evaluative questioning process to the work that you do? How and with whom?

    _____

    _____

_____

_____

6. What kind of courses, groups, or consultation would be valuable to you in the area of professional development and personal growth?

_____

_____

_____

_____

Setting Realistic Personal Standards

1. Write about how you set your own personal standards for the work that you do.

_____

_____

_____

_____

2. Do you choose realistic standards for yourself?

_____

_____

_____

_____

Identifying with Your Work

1. Do you feel connected with your work as a clinician?

_____

_____

_____

_____

2. How do you recognize when you aren't as engaged in your work as you would like to be?

_____

_____

_____

_____

3. What type of program, consultation, course, or retreat would you be interested in to help you to identify more fully with your clinical work?

_____

_____

_____

_____

The Authentic Interview: Our Patients/Clients

Our personal reflections and inner explorations are the groundwork for coming into an authentic clinical interview with our patients. Our own awareness is the best guide that we have in our capacity to be as fully present as possible as we listen to what our patient has to say. As obvious as this may seem, when we pay attention to the subtleties in everyday conversation and can recognize the richness of the nonverbal moments of our interactions, we add another, more personal dimension to our communication. This kind of interaction is helpful for the patient and the clinician as it helps to humanize an often complex and difficult medical setting and creates an appreciation of lived experience. Being accessible, respectful and caring with our patients is an essential foundation for aware and conscious conversation. We need to take our patients' concerns seriously.

It's Really This Simple: The Basics of the Clinical Interview

How Are You?

Communication begins with making contact by simply asking someone, "How are you?" And then, we need to listen to what the person says.

There may be some very real time limits that prevent you from having a lengthy conversation, but when you begin by setting up an atmosphere of interest and caring you create a safe space for people to feel that they have an open avenue of communication. Even taking 5 minutes to acknowledge the person you are with can be enough for them to feel seen and heard. You may discover a great deal about the emotional needs of your patient in these initial contacts, and it is not amiss to ask them if they are interested in psychosocial or psychotherapeutic referrals to help them talk about how they are feeling. Along with your knowledge, bring your understanding that every patient is a unique individual whose life circumstances, cultural background, and personal history affect their lives. We learn about people's lives by being curious about them. We need to ask questions.

Who Are You?

When you ask someone the question, "How are you?" and then listen to what they say you are showing that you are curious about who they are as an individual. It is essential that you are curious about the person who is sitting in front of you. This is the number one instruction I give to people I supervise or consult with, because without bringing your curiosity to an interaction with another human being, you are merely performing the rote duty of taking information about them, not learning who they are. Being engaged and involved in the interactions that you have with your patients conveys to them that you are interested in who they are as another human being, not just a number on a chart. Giving people time, not rushing through the interview, and being patient with them as they may struggle to express themselves, all contribute to satisfying contact between patient and clinician. We need to connect.

What Concerns You?

Concern as it is presented in this book involves both showing your own concern for your patient and helping the patient to locate their own concerns about their well-being. The word *concern* is useful as it is generally not threatening, unlike asking someone how they feel or even what they think, but rather offers a way to reflect on what really matters to them. When you bring concern to your work with patients, you let them know that you take them, yourself, and all that the two of you are dealing with together seriously. Caring for patients means showing authentic concern and bringing compassion into our interactions with them. We need to care.

What Would You Like to Talk About?

It is our responsibility as clinicians to ask our patients what they want and need. I encourage people to share their hopes about what they may want from our interactions. By opening up with a conversational tone, you create a friendly, human dialogue that includes all concerned. Our main task is to listen, to be sure the patient understands what we are saying, and to pay attention to what is not being said as much as the words that are spoken. In essence, it is our responsibility as the clinician to be sure that we are on the same page, particularly during important conversations. We need to listen.

These reminders serve to help us remember that the simple and genuine act of being present with and for another human being, being curious about who they are as a person, and listening to their concerns create a healing connection. For us, as clinicians, this way of being allows us our own humanity, giving us a feeling of connectedness both with our patients and within ourselves. When we feel connected, we are less prone to feeling the emptiness of disconnection that leads to alienation and burnout.

Universal Themes in Cancer Survivorship

The themes discussed next were mentioned in Chapter 2 as the concerns most often reported by cancer survivors on distress screening forms. In this workbook section, we consider them in more depth as a way for you to understand the emotional territory that survivors inhabit. I include this list in a more expanded format as I believe it will help you to listen for and identify these common and very significant issues that your patients will bring up. Depending on your role with your patient, you may chose to delve further into these themes or refer the patient to another clinician who is better suited to attend to these particular needs.

- **Living with uncertainty:** Living with uncertainty is almost always the number one concern that people who are cancer survivors, as well as people who are living with cancer, face on an ongoing basis. Sometimes it is named, but often uncertainty comes disguised as obsessive fear or shows up in searches for some kind of guarantee that illness will not return.

  By recognizing these signs that a patient is struggling with uncertainty and referring the patient to appropriate therapeutic resources, you give them the opportunity to explore these feelings in a more congruous setting for their personal needs. You may want to let them know that you understand and give them the positive message that learning to live with uncertainty may be the greatest challenge as well as the most profound opportunity after drawing the short straw of a life-threatening or chronic illness. You could share with your patients that accepting uncertainty can create a newfound sense of freedom and aliveness if they are willing to meet and explore the challenges of uncertainty after cancer by exploring who they are now in their life.

- **Issues of mortality:** "You're still here." I have used this simple statement time and time again with people who are struggling to believe that they have a future after a cancer diagnosis. It is also effective with those who are living with cancer who, understandably, have difficulty focusing on what lies ahead of them. Following this statement with open-ended questions about interests, passions, or current life events helps to focus the person on the reality of being in the present moment in a pragmatic manner. How do we continue to stay with the present moment while facing the reality of our mortality? When this question is posed as something to explore it opens many doors and windows that lead to the patient discovering what matters to them now in their lives.

- **Identity struggles after cancer:** James Bugental wrote, "What is essential to a meaningful life is a developing sense of personal identity."[12] Cancer survivors may struggle with their identity after they have been a patient or a "sick person." They need guidance in exploring who they are now, and this may often involve recalibrating their wants, needs, and their expectations about themselves, others, and their life. This personal search is not about "Who am I as a cancer patient, and what does being sick mean?" but " Who am I as a person, and what does that mean to me in my life now?" A pithy question to ask someone is, "What matters to you?" Then, just allow them to reflect without the need for "the answer" but remind them that it is the search for what matters that is flexible, ever changing, and unending.

- **Body image issues:** It's important to normalize body image issues so that you can help the patient open up to disclose what they are thinking and feeling. Physical changes may be both temporary and permanent as well as both visible and invisible to others. Regardless of externals, the patient may carry within them distressing and confusing thoughts and feelings about the differences in their body after cancer treatment; this can be very isolating. Men and women have different issues regarding disturbances in their body and appearance, and it's vital to recognize that both genders suffer. Men may focus more on function, physical ability, and personal power as significant identity issues. Women are constantly bombarded with how they should appear (beautiful and thin) and how their appearance is related to their value as a female. However, regardless of the differences, fundamentally body image is really about self-acceptance and self-care and is complex and personal by its very nature.

- **Loss:** Acknowledging the losses that have occurred and helping the patient find their way in the face of how their lives have changed and how they meet the external and internal challenges they have endured and helping them move into acceptance rather than resignation and giving up are key components in survivorship. We can guide them in the exploration of the losses that they may have experienced: fatigue or loss of energy, relationships, fertility/sexuality, body image, self-esteem, work, financial areas, faith, trust, and hope. We can validate the losses that are real for them without sinking into a hopeless or helpless abyss and reassure them that they can mourn old hopes and dreams as they learn to discover new ones.

- **Quality of life:** Quality of life is a phrase used often, particularly in end-of-life care. It's not as featured in survivorship care perhaps because the assumption is, "You made it, you're alive, move on." However, what does quality of life really mean, and how do we help our patients explore what their own quality of life looks like and feels like? The questions included in this workbook are all designed to help the cancer survivor find meaningful ways to connect within themselves so that they may learn how they want to be in their lives—this is quality of life in its most active and engaged form.

- **Anxiety:** Too many times, cancer survivors face a pathologizing attitude about their fears and anxieties. Almost every one of my clients has told me a story of how their anxiety was treated as if there was something wrong with them rather than having the experience of receiving nurturing and accepting feedback. It's scary to have cancer. It's scary not to know when or if you will have a recurrence. It's time to normalize these fears. This does not mean falling into a house of horrors and remaining terrified, it merely means listening to the fears and anxieties because the natural enemy of fear is being listened to and validated while conveying the message that, like any other emotion, it is not permanent and will pass.

- **Depression:** Feelings of depression should be normalized as well as distinguished from feelings of sadness, grief, and loss. Assessing when a patient is clinically depressed as opposed to what is normal considering the situation their cancer diagnosis created is important so that they do not feel ashamed of their emotions. When a cancer survivor is expressing feelings of sadness and grief, rather than giving them a diagnosis of clinical depression and, at times, prescribing antidepressant or antianxiety medication, simply allowing them time and space to process their feelings can help their healing. Referrals to support groups, psychotherapy, workshops, and online resources can all provide needed structures that help cancer survivors move through this next phase of their cancer diagnosis.

- **Self-criticism over emotional responses:** Cancer survivors can fall into a place of self-criticism and self-blame related to the pressures they may feel after finishing treatment. Once they are "set free" from whatever regime they have been following, they can feel out of control, vulnerable, and unsure of how to move forward in their lives. This is another area to recognize and normalize for them in order to help relieve some of the internal and external push to "get over it" and find their "new normal." Letting them know that they do not have to continually be finding deep meaning in their experience with cancer can be tremendously relieving. In essence, give them permission to slow down, rest, and take a deep breath.

When we present the opportunity for authentic transformation to cancer survivors in a manner that does not feel like pressure for them to "get on with it" or be a "good cancer patient" who has a positive attitude and is a "real fighter," we are communicating with them in an empathic and humanistic way. Yet we are still letting them know that, if they choose, they can create a genuine exploration of themselves and their experience, which can be an authentic transformative experience. We need to be clear that this is not necessarily an easy path, that there are no shortcuts, and that the choice is completely an individual endeavor. However, by introducing transformation as a possibility, we give our patients the choice of how they want to heal.

Helping Patients Tell Their Stories

This section corresponds to the workbook templates in *Surviving the Storm: Telling Your Cancer Story* (Krauter, 2017), which is a book you may offer your patients. The following sections in this book serve as a guide for your interviews with patients, their partners, families, and caregivers.

Cancer Survivors

1. How are you? What would you like to talk about?
2. What was it like when you first heard that you had cancer?
3. How was your experience of being in treatment for cancer?
4. How have things been going for you since you finished treatment? Tell me about your experience of finishing treatment for cancer. What stands out for you? What was most helpful, and what was least helpful?
5. Tell me about your experience of living with cancer. What is most helpful and what is least helpful for you as you continue to negotiate your way through treatment?
6. What feelings and concerns do you feel that you carry within you in regard to your diagnosis of cancer?

7. What are your concerns regarding your physical health (for example, is there fatigue or pain, weight issues, sleep problems)?
8. Do you feel listened to by others? Or, do you worry that you are "being a burden" when you talk about your concerns?
9. Do you have financial concerns?
10. How would you say that your life changed after completion of treatment for cancer?
11. What would you say about how your life has changed if you are someone who is living with cancer?
12. Are you hopeful? What do you hope for in your life?
13. What kind of changes have you experienced in your relationships with your partner, your family members, your friends?
14. Do you have concerns about sexuality and intimate relationships?
15. When do you feel worried and scared?
16. What makes you feel relaxed and happy?
17. How do you feel changed by your experience of cancer?
18. When did you feel like a survivor? Or do you?
19. Please tell me what could have been emotionally supportive after finishing treatment.
20. Please tell me what is emotionally supportive if you are living with cancer.
21. What matters to you?

Helping Young Survivors Tell Their Stories

It has only recently been recognized that people under 40 who have been diagnosed with cancer deal with different issues. They often feel left out of survivorship discussions and alienated not only from older survivors but also from their peer group. The following questions are just a brief example of some of the themes that young survivors grapple with in their healing:

1. How are you?
2. What do you want to talk about? Do you feel like people give you the space to talk about your experience?
3. How is your family? Are they anxious about you? How has dealing with your family around your cancer been for you?

4. How is it going in school? Have there been cognitive changes that affect your work?

5. How do you feel that your experience with cancer is affecting your job and career path? What are your concerns?

6. How is it going with your friends and your social network? Do you feel like you fit in? Do the people around you get what you're going through?

7. Do you sometimes feel more mature than your peer group? How does that show up, and what does it feel like to you?

8. Do you feel understood? Who can you talk to?

9. What are your concerns about sexuality? Fertility issues? Do you feel comfortable talking about these concerns and issues? How and when do you decide to bring them up?

10. What's it like to deal with your physical changes and challenges, like fatigue, scarring, losses, and other ways in which your body has been affected by cancer and treatments? How does this affect your self-image?

11. What's it like to be at a place in your life where you may need to depend more on your family when you want to become more independent and start your own life?

12. What happens when you have been out on your own and need to return home to get the help and support you need?

13. What are your biggest worries and fears?

14. What makes you happy and relaxed?

15. How do you feel changed by your experience?

16. When did you feel like a survivor? Or do you?

17. What is your experience of being someone who is living with cancer?

18. Tell me what you wish for yourself.

Notes

1. Jack Coulehan, MD, Take Off Your Clothes [Poetry and Medicine]. *JAMA*. 2016; 315(6):615.

2. Carl Faber, PhD, *On Listening*, Perseus Press, New York, 1976, p. 3.

3. Atul Gawande, MD, Big Med [Annals of Health Care]. *The New Yorker*, August 13, 2012, p. 18.

4. Cheryl Strayed, *Brave Enough*, Knopf, New York, 2015, p. 14.

5. James F. T. Bugental, PhD, *The Art of the Psychotherapist*, Norton, New York, 1987, p. 238.

6. Bugental, *Art of the Psychotherapist*, p. 221.

7. Bugental, *Art of the Psychotherapist*, p. 202.

8. James F. T. Bugental, *The Search for Authenticity*, Irvington, New York, 1981, p. 102.

9. Robert Frost, A Time to Talk, in *Mountain Interval*, Holt, New York, 1920, p. 44.

10. Bugental, *Search for Authenticity*, p. 452.

11. Bugental, *Art of the Psychotherapist*, p. 7.

12. Bugental, *Art of the Psychotherapist*, p. 228.

CHAPTER 4 — A Conversation of Hope and Healing

Cultural Humility

Before you learn the tender gravity of kindness,
you must travel where the Indian in a white poncho
lies dead by the side of the road.
You must see how this could be you,
how he too was someone
who journeyed through the night with plans
and the simple breath that kept him alive.

—Naomi Shihab Nye, "Kindness"[1]

In 1975, just 6 years after the Watts riots in Los Angeles, I worked as part of a team at the University of California at Los Angeles (UCLA) Extension called the Arts Neighborhood Development Program. Our goal was to bring visual and performing artists who were of different cultures, race, gender identities, and class together using art as a way to open a conversation of hope and healing. The intention was to use visual and performing arts to tap into the creativity and wisdom of different communities and build relationships between people whose paths were unlikely to cross in day-to-day life.

It's important to acknowledge that I was the only "white girl" on this team, 24 years old, and relatively naïve to the complexities we were attempting to bridge. To this day, I remember what it felt like to walk into one of the workshops offered at this event and to be the only white person in the group. The racial tension in Los Angeles at that time was at an all-time high, and neither I nor anyone else in this group spoke to my presence in this workshop or acknowledged the tension palpable in that room when I walked in.

Now, 41 years later, as a psychotherapist working in cancer healthcare, I find that this kind of dialogue around racial and health disparities is still largely missing among those of us who provide services to cancer patients and cancer survivors. My own private practice was barren of any diversity for decades, and I have long considered the lack of attention to this homogeneity to be a hidden shortcoming in the field of psychology. It wasn't until I began working in Oakland, California, that my private work shifted into more of a multicultural mode. But it is important to note that I am the exception rather than the norm in psychotherapeutic practice.

Long before the term *cultural humility* existed, my initiation into its complexities occurred in 1970 when the University of California at Irvine went on strike to protest the Kent State shootings. In the alternative university that was created during the strike, I attended a class taught by the artist Ed Bereal, whose fierce presence and bold confrontation of racial injustice ripped apart my assumptions, opened my mind, and started my own lifelong course of learning how to be inquisitive, curious, and honest in explorations around race, culture, class, and identity. Now, 46 years later, I include the concerns of cultural humility in this book as an essential part of clinical focus for all of us in cancer healthcare. It is essential that we be curious about the backgrounds of our patients so that we may be as effective and fully present as possible in our relationships with them.

This chapter also could not exist without the many brave writers and academics who've voiced truths about racism, classism, sexism, homophobia, and all other discriminations against other human beings. We all stand on the shoulders of the work they have done, and continue to do, to bring awareness to conscious and unconscious forms of bias.

A 2016 article, "The Association Between Income and Life Expectancy in the United States, 2001–2014," in the *Journal of the American Medical Association* (*JAMA*), reported "that while the importance of the relationship between income and life expectancy is well established, it remains 'poorly understood.'" The research findings in the study stated: "In the United States between 2001 and 2014 higher income was associated with greater longevity, and differences in life expectancy across income groups increased over time."[2] I was struck by the fact that the study went on to report that the association between life expectancy and income varied, and that differences in longevity across income groups decreased in some areas and increased in others. This absolute lack of clarity showcases the complexity of culture, even within a culture that may be construed as homogeneous. The variances speak to the error of generalizing a group of individuals by placing them all together into an undifferentiated mass, as well as addressing the importance of being cautious about depending on stereotypes to define others. The study concluded that the differences in life expectancy were correlated with health behaviors and local area characteristics, which were also race- and class-related. The findings are listed next.

The Association Between Income and Life Expectancy in the United States, 2001–2014

In a groundbreaking analysis of US income and mortality data since 2001, researchers report that:

- Life expectancy at age 40 increases continuously with income percentile.
- The wealthiest 1% have a life expectancy at age 40 that's 10–15 years greater than the poorest 1%.
- The rise in life expectancy associated with income becomes much smaller above a household income of about $200,000.
- Expected age at death for 40-year-olds increased for people in the top income quartile at a rate about 2.5 times that for people in the bottom income quartile.
- Life expectancy at age 40 differs by location, favoring New York and California for people in the bottom income quartile and Utah and Maine for those in the top income quartile.
- Most of the difference in life expectancy between the wealthiest and poorest seems attributable to health behaviors.[3]

The final bullet point in the material from this article appears to suggest that it is "health behavior" that is mostly responsible for the difference in life expectancy from individual to individual even though the findings of the study clearly pointed to wealth disparity as a major factor. While behavior is certainly a key component in health, "good" health behavior is influenced by what is accessible to people. People with low incomes, who do not have access to quality care and to whom healthy food or the components of a "healthy lifestyle" are not available or affordable, have limited choices regarding health behaviors. These same people may not have the option to take time off when they are sick because to do so would incur severe financial consequences. Behavior is often predicated as much on options as it is on choice. Dolores Morehead, Patient Navigator, Women's Cancer Resource Center, told me the following in an oral interview on July 22, 2016:

People have different needs, sometimes invisible and not understood. For example, patients who do not show up for appointments are often looked upon as irresponsible or as having non-compliant behavior. But what if they don't have any transportation or any money to take the bus? What if they don't have childcare? You don't know what their problems are. How do we help them realize that their life is worth it, that they are worthy?

It is essential that we, as clinicians in cancer healthcare, open up and deepen conversations that acknowledge the reality that we inhabit and coexist within a complex and diverse world that includes people of different races, sexual orientation, gender, and class. This is not about a "fix," as there are no easy answers. There is no simple solution that moves us forward from centuries of history, scripted beliefs, and biased behaviors, but at the same time it is no longer acceptable to stand in silence and avoid a dive into the hazardous terrain of diversity and cultural humility.

This chapter does not pretend to be a comprehensive piece on cultural humility. However, my hope is that the information presented and the resources provided will lead you to your own self-inquiry, bring attention to your awareness of yourself and those around you, and encourage a commitment to a lifelong learning process of cultural humility. This commitment involves an ongoing exploration of reflection and expressive questioning, honest self-evaluation, a capacity to engage in demanding and arduous dialogue, and an openness to change.

The fact that we are here and that we speak these words is an attempt to break that silence and bridge some of those differences between us, for it is not difference which immobilizes us, but silence and there are so many silences to break.

—Audre Lorde, "When the Silence Shatters"[4]

In their groundbreaking 1998 editorial, "Cultural Humility Versus Cultural Competence," Melanie Tervalon, MD, MPH, and Jann Murray-Garcia, MD, MPH, wrote the following:

The traditional notion of competence in clinical training as a detached mastery of a theoretically finite body of knowledge may not be appropriate for this area of physician education. Cultural humility is proposed as a more suitable goal in multicultural medical education. Cultural humility incorporates a lifelong commitment to self-evaluation and self-critique, to redressing the power imbalances in the patient-physician dynamic, and to developing mutually beneficial and non-paternalistic clinical advocacy partnerships with communities on behalf of individuals and defined populations.[5]

This seminal editorial aimed at physician training in multicultural education has served as the basis for the ongoing exploration of cultural humility and is referred to in most of the documents and training materials that have followed its publication nearly two decades ago. In this piece, Tervalon and Murray-Garcia proposed that the traditional approach of having some form of mastery or competence in working with people of different cultures may not be the most thorough or effective way to educate clinicians. Their concept of cultural humility was born out of the idea that lifelong learning does not by its very nature have a finite point of competence. They believe that providing ongoing multicultural education in healthcare is the road to a better understanding of the complex and ever-changing issues inherent in diverse populations. In other words, the opinion that we reach a static state of competence in understanding multicultural and class issues can create a false sense of security in having "just enough" knowledge of the issues of diversity to actually perpetuate stereotypes rather than shift perceptions. A person's stance of being "competent enough" implies a level of understanding that is finite and complete rather than holding a perspective of keeping an open mind and heart to the person you are with.

In their article, "Cultural Humility: Essential Foundation for Clinical Researchers," Katherine A. Yeager, PhD, RN, and Susan Bauer-Wu, PhD, RN, FAAN, reported that "how we approach the many factors that contribute to health disparities and social inequities requires an examination of the environment, context, and culture of those experiencing disparities."[6] These researchers reported that in the process of forming a stance of cultural humility, we must examine our personal and cultural beliefs and values around race, ethnicity, class, religion, immigration status, gender roles, ages, linguistic capability, and sexual orientation. The report also states that where people live or grew up matters (i.e., rural, suburban, affluent, or impoverished area) and shapes their views of others. Be mindful that the neighborhood where you live, work, or commute to influences your thoughts, feelings, and values and has an impact on how you define what community means. All of these factors are important points to recognize, explore, and reflect on.

As I read, researched, and reviewed the literature on cultural competence and cultural humility, I was struck by the fact that the bulk of the material has been presented by people of color, which brought questions to my mind. Where are the thoughts and comments of the white population, and how do we (or don't we) participate in these conversations? The absence of a truly multicultural dialogue speaks to people's tendency to turn away from uncomfortable discussions, to have a fear of confrontation, and to possess an unconscious collective shame and guilt that is carried within the dominant culture. In their study, "Measures of Cultural Competence: Examining Hidden Assumptions," Kumas-Tan and coworkers

systematically reviewed the most frequently used cultural competence measures and identified assumptions embedded in these measures: culture is usually equivalent to ethnicity and race, and little attention is given to components of culture such as gender, class, geographic location, country of origin, or sexual preference. These instruments assume that culture is possessed by the patient or the client or the "other." In many of the measures, whiteness is understood and represented as the norm.[7]

But what is "the norm" and what beliefs, assumptions, and experiences are we looking at? *JAMA* published "Racial Bias in Health Care and Health: Challenges and Opportunities," which included this statement:

Some physicians are unaware that racial disparities exist and question the evidence of disparities. Successfully addressing the possibility of clinician bias begins with the awareness of the pervasiveness of disparities, the ways in which bias can influence clinician decision making and behavior, and a commitment to acquiring skills to minimize these processes.[8]

Consider the list that follows: What thoughts and feelings come up for you when you look at these categories that list where biases exist? Which ones do you identify with? Bring your awareness of your personal experience as you spend time with these points.

- Race
- Ethnicity
- Class
- Religion
- Immigration status
- Gender roles
- Age
- Language
- Sexual orientation
- Disability

In order to move through these ancient and strongly held beliefs, we must let go of blame and fault-finding. Change and transformation cannot come about in an atmosphere of blame. Blaming another person (or an entire group of people) merely continues to perpetuate the "us-versus-them" mentality of separation and, ultimately, an ignorance of the complexities of our world and the multitude of human beings living on this planet. The conversation we're engaging in here concerns the transformation of our clinical work with patients and the collaboration between all of us as clinicians. This dialogue is not only about humanizing the clinician–patient relationship, but also about forming collegial connections that allow for satisfying exchanges between clinicians. Too often, a hierarchical structure in healthcare imposes distance, and even marginalization, in communication between clinicians.

Clinicians have shared with me their own experiences of frustration with this lack of communication due to assumed (and assigned) power roles. I remember when my father was ill and how the hands-on health aides in his facility, and not the physician who saw him infrequently, were the ones who provided me with the most dependable updates on his condition. In fact, it's the rare physician who acknowledges the benefits of the hands-on, personal information that an aide or a nurse could provide not only to the family of a patient but also to the treating physician.

A psychotherapist friend of mine who specializes in cancer health-care told me once that she has experienced great resistance from physicians around giving information that could be helpful in her work with patients. And it is well known that oncology nurses in the infusion rooms are the people patients are told to turn to for support and advice, yet these same nurses often feel marginalized by the physicians they work with. These are only a few brief examples of the kinds of power struggles that can occur in the culture of the helping profession, which dehumanizes clinicians by placing them into hierarchical and stereotypical roles.

One antidote to this kind of power struggle is the encouragement of personal encounters. Allowing others to tell their stories so that we can learn who they really are and being willing to be vulnerable enough to share our own stories is a way of being a part of a conversation of hope and healing. Each one of us has a unique tale and the need to be witnessed as we tell our story. We all create stories about others in our own minds based on nothing more than impressions gained without any actual experience. These are assumptive stories, not true stories told to us by another person, whose experience then becomes real and understandable once we have listened to them. We cannot continue to depend on the dangerous and shameful practice of relying on incomplete second-hand accounts of another person or a group of people, or an entire culture, as a way to understand both our differences and our similarities. In her 2009 TED talk, "The Danger of a Single Story," author Chimamanda Ngozi Adichie said: "Show a people as only one thing and that is what they become."[9]

Personal Awareness

Awareness begins with the work we do within ourselves. A commitment to self-reflection, curiosity, finding the courage to speak up, the ability to ask questions, and the willingness to admit ignorance are all powerful ways to learn. Uncertainty is a sign of humility, and humility is the ability or the willingness to learn and the openness to have difficult conversations. Living with uncertainty means accepting that we don't ever reach a point of completely knowing ourselves or others and is a major step in the understanding of the complexities of cultural humility. Yeager and Bauer-Wu stated: "An individual's culture is not a single identity; rather it's a rich mixture of many influences and values. Thus understanding oneself and others is a complex and lifelong process."[10]

Exploring our own culture is not one dimensional because most of us, particularly in the United States, are a mixture of different backgrounds and cultural combinations. I grew up not knowing until I was well into my forties that my paternal great-grandmother was American Indian. This family secret had been held by my paternal grandmother for her entire life. I would later learn, through letters and from various relatives, that this was due to her shame of being mistreated as a "half-breed."

There are countless examples of people like my grandmother who've had to hide their true experiences or who've passed the shame of who they are on to subsequent generations. With the brutal history of the discrimination of people of color, the LGBT (lesbian, gay, bisexual, transgender) community, and all of those from different classes and cultures, it makes sense that past generations tried to hide their identities in order to ensure their survival.

Fast forward to the present and we find that people are wanting to be seen for who they are; they want to be recognized and valued as human beings with diverse cultural and class backgrounds. They certainly don't want to be lumped into a generic category that assumes that all members of their particular group are identical. Yeager and Bauer stated: "Minority groups such as American Indians, Alaska Natives, African Americans, Hispanics, Asians, or Pacific Islanders are often given cultural characteristics, but those descriptions can miss the mark. Within each group, many subpopulations exist with very different cultures, historical experiences, and views on health and illness."[11] This is true regardless of whichever group we identify with, and it stresses the importance of continued commitment to self-awareness as well as an openness to those who may be labeled different from us.

A constantly evolving awareness of our own bias requires that we listen well to our thoughts and feelings and pay attention to the words that we speak. It means that we engage with others who come from different backgrounds to discover not only our differences but also what we share in common. Personal awareness is the essence of cultural humility as it demands openness and honesty of each of us; when we bring those qualities to our interactions, we can create an unfolding dialogue between one another.

Professional Awareness

I went with my mother to her oncology appointment and was asking some questions about her diagnosis and treatment. At one point the oncologist swiveled around in his chair and pointed at the medical degree behind his desk saying, "Do you have one of these, (pointing again) do you have one of these?" I replied, "No, but I have been in the field of cancer healthcare long enough that I advocate for older women. I can advocate for my mom.

—Dolores Morehead, Patient Navigator, Women's Cancer Resource Center, oral interview, July 22, 2016

In our profession, we need to be aware of the power imbalances inherent in our roles as clinicians. Attention to power dynamics between us and our patients is vital for a healing relationship that is person centered. The consciousness of how power plays a part in our professional roles with other colleagues is often less clear and can be acted out in varying degrees of invalidation and marginalization between clinicians. Regardless of role or position, respectful communication needs to be seen as a basic requirement in our relationships with our patients as well as with our colleagues. We can unwittingly treat others insensitively when we assign them to roles that correspond with race, class, and gender. Cultural humility calls on us to explore and identify our unconscious biases so that we can be respectful and sensitive to the person we are with. These biases are insidious for they have deep and tangled roots that are not easy to dig up and lay aside in favor of an open perspective, but as clinicians we have a responsibility to do this gardening work in order to better serve others. A continual emphasis on the principles of cultural humility, ongoing discussion, groups, workshops, and open conversations that ask questions rather than make assumptions are all part of developing these skills and are part of the lifelong learning process. Learning to listen to ourselves and to others in order to catch subtle biases and attitudes is an ongoing process.

Almost four decades ago, when I had just started my counseling internship, I was talking with my clinical supervisor, freaked out and feeling like I didn't know what I was doing when I sat with my clients. She calmly replied to me, "You must never stop questioning what you are doing and who you are to sit in that chair. If you ever stop questioning yourself, you may as well leave the field." This statement speaks not only to humility, but also to what the Zen Buddhist tradition calls beginner's mind. In each interaction we have, we are beginners, regardless of how many years we have worked as clinicians. Each clinical interview is different because we are creating a unique relationship with every individual that we meet. In my book *Surviving the Storm: A Workbook for Telling Your Cancer Story* (Krauter, 2017), I wrote about learning to live with uncertainty. Cancer survivors must embrace what they don't, or can't, know. Because uncertainty is part of life experience, it's valuable for practitioners to develop ways to speak to the myriad aspects of uncertainty in the work we do. We begin anew with each patient every day.

Our sensitivity to another human being is part of being respectful toward others. Like respect, sensitivity is both a basic and a universal truth in communication. The art of humanistic work and the understanding of relational skills transcends differences and brings forth what is fundamental for human contact and understanding. Ongoing attention to personal awareness helps us, as clinicians, to identify the shadow of power and our unconscious assumptions, which then results in the building of a strong, healing alliance in our work with patients and our collaboration with colleagues.

Community Awareness

In July 2015, I attended the International Psycho-Oncology/American Psychosocial Oncology (IPOS) World Conference, in Washington, DC. Nearly 1,000 people from 29 countries gathered to discuss the vital importance of implementing quality psychosocial care for cancer patients and their communities. In her plenary address at this conference, Luzia

Travado, PhD, President, International Psycho-Oncology Society, stated that:

The International Psycho-Oncology Society (IPOS) Human Rights Task Force has been working since 2008 to raise awareness and support from within IPOS and the IPOS Federation for the relevance of Psychosocial Cancer Care as a Human Rights issue. We seek to advocate for this issue internationally and nationally through existing Human Rights laws.

At that conference, I listened to many stories around the need to attend to the human right to healthcare in this world. I heard about children in Kenya who are kept in the hospital until their families can pay the bill for the treatment they have received. I now know that many people with terminal cancer die extremely painful deaths because they do not have palliative care medications to ease their suffering. In Kenya, caregivers will be punished for allowing families to receive the bodies of their loved ones if they have not completed payment for their treatment. Other such atrocities occur daily and are endured silently on the planet. Many are denied not only quality physical treatment but also attention to the emotional and social trauma of a cancer diagnosis. Due to the healthcare system in the United States, a serious medical diagnosis is the most common reason for bankruptcy. Cancer survivors in Australia, unsatisfied with the quality of emotional care, rebelled and have formed highly successful peer support groups. They became advocates for their own care as well as the care of other cancer survivors. As consumers, they raised their voices, and the government as well as the medical establishment listened. As a powerful patient group, they brought about change in the system. They did not remain silent.

It is our responsibility as clinicians to have knowledge of the community in which we work. We are responsible for providing advocacy for community organizations and educating ourselves about people and their practices in our community rather than remaining solely in our offices or medical centers. We can ask about people's beliefs, and by doing so we come to have better understanding, respect, and acceptance of others. I carry a story with me about a young Latina woman patient advocate working in the United States who worked with a woman dying of cancer. The patient's cultural and religious beliefs did not allow for dying and death to be openly spoken of. Indeed, the patient and her family denied the impending death entirely. However, there were children involved who would need to be raised after this woman's death. So the patient advocate, while respecting the needs of the family to deny the mother's imminent death, was able to locate an aunt in Latin America who was willing to take the children; the patient advocate arranged to bring this woman to the United States before her niece died.

To the very end, no one spoke of death, but after their mother died, the children were taken by the aunt back to her country in Latin America and not placed in the childcare system because they did not have family who were able to care for them in the United States. For me, this story unfolds as a beautiful example of following the needs of the patient while also taking clinical and ethical responsibility for the needs of others. In many ways, this case follows in the tradition of many Hispanic cultures, where family involvement is often a critical aspect in the healthcare of the cancer patient. However, there are common barriers to quality care that include language and immigration status, which cannot be denied. Sensitivity to religious practices is also crucial as well as attention to the often traditional male and female roles in the Latin culture.

In 2015, I attended a workshop with other clinicians; one Latina woman spoke with emotion about the fact that the only other Latino people in that facility were cleaning rooms and waiting tables. She felt disenfranchised and was brave in stating her truth. Fortunately, the group attending the workshop took this in, and we had a conversation that not only made her feel part of the group but also helped the rest of us become more conscious of her experience of being a person of color.

Another important group to consider in the conversation of cultural humility is the LGBT community. In 2009, Lambda Legal conducted a survey with the help of over one hundred partner organizations as part of a national Health Care Fairness Campaign that was the first to examine the disparities and bias surrounding the LGBT and HIV communities and how these prejudices lead to barriers of health care. In this study, people who identified as transgender or gender-nonconforming reported experiencing the highest rates of discrimination and barriers to care as compared with those who reported discrimination based on sexual orientation or HIV status. The study went on to report: "More than other groups, transgender or gender-nonconforming respondents experience alienation from the healthcare system. Overall, nearly 90 percent of TGNC [transgender/nonconforming] respondents experienced one or more barriers to care."[12] The LGBT group is beginning to be better recognized in cancer healthcare, but there are still unconscious biases from which we cannot close our eyes.

Yet another group that is often quieter and sometimes harder to acknowledge is the group of people with disabilities. I have spoken with people who have obvious disabilities as well as with those who have hidden disabilities; both groups tell me that they often feel ignored to the point of not "being on the radar." With hidden disabilities, there is the obvious fact that these issues are largely invisible and even sometimes denied as "only psychosomatic" and therefore not real. For those whose disabilities are often disturbing for others to see or be around, the theme of being isolated from others, where they are not visible to others, is extremely painful and costly to the quality of life for the disabled individual.

As clinicians, we can learn to advocate with humility; we can open ourselves to learning about different communities and organizations with respect, sensitivity, and curiosity so that we may weave together the threads of different neighborhoods and societies in a pattern of understanding and acceptance. All the stories and reports that I have shared have a common theme—the benefits of opening up a conversation between people.

Institutional Awareness

Cassandra Falby, LMFT, Program Director at Women's Cancer Resource Center, told me a story of a homeless woman in treatment for cancer having to spend the night in a shelter who had difficulty getting to treatment and who even struggled to find a way of being treated for her cancer. In an oral interview on June 3, 2016, Cassandra said:

There are people who have to 'piece it together' in a time when they are very ill and I feel disappointment in the systems that exist, the inadequate community resources, and the lack of communication between community agencies. It helps to be able to offer alternatives.

The challenges of institutional racism and biased attitudes toward diverse demographics runs deep and wide. The occurrence of healthcare disparities is a prime and horrifying example of the need for change within our healthcare system. Questions, conversations, confrontations, and advocacy for change are essential in order to shift what is so embedded into the system that we sometimes can't discern the difficulties that need to be addressed. Tervalon and Murray-Garcia wrote: "The same processes expected to affect change in physician trainees should simultaneously exist in the institutions whose agenda is to develop cultural competence through educational programs."[13]

There are important questions that require the same self-reflective and self-evaluative explorations at an institutional level as those asked of a responsible individual clinician. Indeed, many clinicians, like Cassandra Falby and myself, have been daunted by the depth of institutional racism. My own experiences have occurred in more than one survivorship committee assigned the task of planning quality survivorship care. I designed what I believed to be a well-thought-out, sensitive, and deep program for the emotional support of those who had been diagnosed with and treated for cancer. In both instances, the initial response of the others involved was not only favorable but also enthusiastic, so I continued to work on these programs. However, when it was time to put the survivorship programs into action, the bulk of my program was ignored or cut because it was considered "too sophisticated for our demographic," and the belief was that we should reorganize the material to fit a "fifth-grade level" of intelligence and experience. The members of the committee in charge of implementing the survivorship program put a different program into place, and soon after this decision, these committees disbanded.

The conversation about institutional racism, which includes all forms of discrimination, is perhaps the most difficult to open up, much less stay with during the inevitable tension-filled moments that will be present. The barriers to insisting on institutional accountability seem too high and wide to break through, and all too often we give up because we feel inadequate to the task; we turn away from the tough questions, we remain silent. We get stuck looking for easy solutions to complex problems; we try to find answers to questions rather than investigating the questions themselves.

In our linear, limited scope of thinking, we give more credence to simple answers and avoid exploring more thoroughly that which we don't understand. We need to look back through centuries into the bias and discrimination we have denied so we do not carry it further into the future. Similar to the foundation of transpersonal (beyond the personal) psychology, looking at institutional racism demands we move beyond our personal perspective to explore the issues of power and privilege that are embedded in healthcare institutions.

We don't want people to fall into the system—they may never be seen again. How are institutions training their staff in regard to cultural humility?

—Cassandra Falby, LMFT, oral interview June 30, 2016

The questions that follow were composed by Melanie Tervalon and Jann Murray-Garcia; they are excellent examples of topics and themes to explore when looking at bringing cultural humility into institutions. They could certainly have many applications in training clinicians in cultural humility.

List of Questions by Tervalon and Murray-Garcia

- What is the demographic profile of the faculty?
- Is the faculty composition inclusive of members from diverse cultural, racial, ethnic, and sexual orientation backgrounds?
- Are faculty members required to undergo multicultural training as are the youngest students of the profession?
- Does the institution support inclusion and respectful, substantive discussions of the clinical implications of difference?
- What institutional processes contradict or obstruct lessons taught and learned in a multicultural curriculum?
- What is the history of the healthcare institution with the surrounding community?
- What present model of relationship between the institution and the community is seen by the trainees?[14]

What's it like for the clinician not to understand the language, the culture?

—Cassandra Falby, LMFT, oral interview, June 30, 2016

Language barriers are not only about language, but also about being clear and using words that are understandable rather than using medical or psychological terms that dehumanize the conversation. Talking in jargon that is exclusive and using acronyms rather than full names are ways we can alienate and isolate or inadvertently showcase our own power or superiority. In an oral interview on June 23, 2016, with Cheryl Jones, LMFT, she told me, "Doctors need to understand when people don't understand them." When we are trained to listen well and observe the person we are speaking with, we notice when they don't understand. Their eyes may look glassy, or they may stare blankly back at us. There is a feeling in the room the other person isn't quite there with us. These are all simple signs that we have "lost our audience" and need to check in. Falby brought up a great point by asking what it's like for the clinician not to know or understand the language or culture of their patient. This may be something clinicians don't ask themselves, and yet we should— always. There's a somewhat simple solution to this problem, after all. Ask your patients about themselves, their values and beliefs, where they come from, and who they are as a human being. Using the language of the heart, we enter a relationship open and ready to receive the person as they are, not as we expect them to be.

Ethnocentrism, which holds a belief of superiority in relationship to either a personal ethnic group or different racial, religious, gender groups, suggests that there are problems because we are different and often implies that individuals as well as entire societal groups and cultures are inferior. Basically, ethnocentrism judges another person or culture by the values and beliefs of their own culture. This stance is more common than any of us like to acknowledge, both within ourselves and with others. When stereotypical misunderstanding and labeling replaces the hard work of digging deep into who you are and who the other person is, we continue to create and perpetuate bias. However, if we break the silence to have a conversation of the heart and mind, we stand a chance of learning about one another in a respectful, sensitive, and humane manner. It is within an authentic relationship that we can know one another and move past assumptions and stereotypes to know and understand rather than judge and assume.

We cannot pretend that disparities in healthcare don't exist anymore as this denial is only indicative of how embedded these inequities are within ourselves, our communities, and our institutions. The failure to recognize bias and disparities continues to make suffering and illness other forms of violence. We need to highlight the uncomfortable aspects of racism, sexism, homophobia, and all other discrimination against those we deem different and advocate for a change in attitude in regard to quality of healthcare for these groups. We need to find the courage to speak of these inequities as we find new paths to fresh answers and new solutions to long-standing problems.

Attending an occasional evening lecture or taking a weekend workshop or a seminar for continuing education requirements is not the answer to an ongoing commitment to cultural humility. Mastering an art takes decades, and while a level of mastery in cultural humility can be achieved through similar discipline and practice, in reality lifelong learning remains an alive and continual process without an end point. If someone claims to have reached mastery or a level of cultural competence, beware.

The narrative storytelling process presented in both my books (*Surviving the Storm* and this volume) can be used effectively to open a person-centered conversation on cultural humility. By utilizing a relational framework, we foster a mindful, self-reflective, and self-aware dialogue that can help us access our humanity as we traverse the rocky path of breaking the silence of ancient discrimination so that we may move into an era of cultural humility. The workbook section that follows on cultural humility is designed to help you explore your own thoughts and feelings as well as aid you in finding ways to incorporate a mindful approach to the important issues of culture in your clinical practice.

According to Title VI of the Civil Rights Act (1964), services provided with funding from the federal government must be delivered without regard to race, color, or national origin.

Of all the forms of inequality, injustice in health care is the most shocking and inhumane.

—Martin Luther King, Jr.[15]

While it is important to learn about health beliefs and practices of different cultures, equating cultural competence with simply having completed a past series of training sessions is an inadequate and potentially harmful model of professional development.

—Melanie Tervalon, Cultural Humility Training of Trainers, 2015[16]

Cultural competency says, "I'm the expert." Cultural humility says, "You're the expert." As clinicians, we need to respect and interact with patients from diverse backgrounds. This requires a personal awareness of our own biases and the ways in which we are ignorant of the experiences, beliefs, and values of those who come from different backgrounds. Bringing curiosity to clinical interviews and opening up personal conversations are avenues of understanding the people we are working with. These types of interactions inform us about not only the patient but also the types of health behaviors that may be particular to that person's culture. It is our responsibility to be curious and attentive to different worldviews in our clinical work with cancer survivors. It is vital that we move beyond the classic (Western culture) definition of white, heterosexual, English-speaking, and Judeo-Christian individuals as "normal."

How to Approach Your Patients

Keep in mind that the human contact we have with our patients creates a healing relationship. When we allow ourselves to make an authentic connection with others, not only do we gain important knowledge about their backgrounds, but also we give ourselves an opportunity to show our own humanity. The following suggestions can help you to structure clinical interviews that include the values of cultural humility:

- See your patients as capable human beings with distinct personal histories
- View the relationship with your patients as collaborative
- Be willing to learn from your patients

- Take risks by asking questions and acknowledging what you don't know or understand
- Ask open-ended questions
- Don't make assumptions
- Agree to disagree respectfully
- Listen
- Listen
- Listen

These simple guidelines can help you to create a dialogue of curiosity and acceptance. It's important to look at conversations with your patients as beginnings, "ice breakers" to support ongoing conversations you will have with them for the duration of your relationship. We can't cover every inch of the multicultural ground that lies before us in one, or even two, meetings, but we can set the stage for continued learning over time.

Modes of Learning Cultural Humility

You may be wondering how you can find resources for learning the principles and practices of cultural humility. Beyond the written and spoken words on the complexities of the subject, the list that follows suggests different modes that can be utilized for multicultural education. If your facility or institution does not provide this type of learning experience, you may want to consider contacting some of the resources in this book as well as organizing your own curriculum with other interested clinicians.

- Classes, workshops, trainings, evening lectures
- Ongoing small-group discussions
- Guest lectures and discussions with multicultural presenters
- Education on self-reflection, self-critique, and honest self-evaluation
- Resources for the practice of self-awareness for clinicians
- Education on person-centered communication as it applies to cultural/class issues
- Experiential training on interview skills with diverse populations

Developing Awareness in Cultural Humility

The following sections are designed for your personal reflection as well as for use in conversation with your patients and your colleagues.

Personal Awareness

1. How much do you know about your own cultural background?

---

2. What class background do you identify with?

---

3. Does your clinical practice involve working with a diverse population? What types of experiences have you had?

---

4. What kinds of messages did you get from your family when you were around people who were different from you?

---

5. Self-reflect on your attitudes around culture and class. What do you notice? Do you find yourself censoring attitudes that are "politically incorrect"?

_____

_____

_____

_____

6. Do you have an awareness of your personal biases? How do you notice them? When do they come up?

_____

_____

_____

_____

7. Have you ever been in a situation where discriminatory language or behavior occurred? What happened for you? Did you speak up? Did you feel unable to speak up?

_____

_____

_____

_____

8. Do you have a self-reflective practice regarding your personal biases? Describe it.

_____

_____

_____

_____

9. Reflect on and write about ways in which you can bring a reflective, honest, and evaluative approach to your work with diverse populations.

_____

_____

_____

_____

Professional Awareness

1. Does your work involve a multicultural element? How would you describe your experience?

_____

_____

_____

_____

2. Do you have colleagues whose backgrounds differ from your own?

_____

_____

_____

_____

3. Have you experienced power dynamics as a professional in healthcare? Are you aware of when you may become caught in a hierarchical role with your patients?

_____

_____

_____

_____

4. Do you feel that you have an adequate education in cultural humility? How much attention has been paid to that part of your clinical work?

_____

_____

_____

_____

5. Do you have opportunities for professional dialogues around issues of culture and class? What would you like to see offered in this area of your profession?

_____

_____

_____

_____

6. In what ways do you challenge yourself and your knowledge around diversity?

_____

_____

_____

_____

7. Describe how you remain open to understanding and learning about those who come from a different background from your own.

_____

_____

_____

_____

Community Awareness

1. Are you involved with the community that you serve?

_____

_____

_____

_____

2. Do you have relationships with other agencies and organizations in your community?

_____

_____

_____

_____

3. How do you feel about being an advocate for those you serve?

_____

_____

_____

_____

4. Do you have an adequate resource and referral system in your community? What needs do you see in this area?

_____

_____

_____

_____

Institutional Awareness

1. If you work in an institution, do you feel that there is adequate attention to themes of diversity?

   _____

   _____

   _____

   _____

2. Does your institution mirror the intentions of personal awareness that include reflection, critique, honest evaluation, and openness?

   _____

   _____

   _____

   _____

3. If you work in the private sector, do you feel that your own work environment takes the intentions of cultural humility into consideration?

   _____

   _____

   _____

   _____

4. Do you think that the demographic of the staff in the institution represents a multicultural group?

   _____

   _____

   _____

   _____

5. Have you experienced discrimination in an institutional setting? Tell what happened.

   _____

   _____

6. Does your institution or your professional organization offer opportunities for multicultural education?

_____

_____

_____

_____

7. Do you feel that institutions in cancer healthcare bring attention to the issues of cultural humility in the form of policies and requirements?

_____

_____

_____

_____

You can make use of these questions to open a deeper exploration of the conversation of cultural humility. These are messy dialogues, meaning that mistakes will be made, toes might be stepped on, and feelings could be hurt. But if we bring an openness to listening and learning from one another, and include the practice of forgiveness when we unintentionally stumble, we can begin to unpack the bags of bias. It's a start.

On the deepest level, problems such as racism, war and starvation are not solved by economics and politics alone. Their source is prejudice and fear in the human heart—and their solution also lies in the human heart. What the world needs most is people who are less bound by prejudice. It needs more love, more generosity, more mercy, more openness. The root of human problems is not a lack of resources but comes from the misunderstanding, fear, and separateness that can be found in the hearts of people.

—Jack Kornfield[17]

Notes

1. Naomi Shahib Nye, Kindness, *Words Under the Words: Selected Poems*, Eighth Mountain Press, Portland, OR, 1995, pp. 42–43. Copyright © 1995.

2. Raj Chetty, PhD, Michael Stepner, BA, Sarah Abraham, BA, et al., The Association Between Income and Life Expectancy in the United States, 2001–2014. *JAMA*. 2016;315(16):1750. doi:10.1001/jama.2016.

3. Chetty et al., Association Between Income and Life Expectancy, p. 1763. Reprinted with permission from the Copyright Clearance Center.

4. Audre Lorde, When the Silence Shatters: Post-Black Women's Truth and Reconciliation Commission, Reflections from a Testifier, Ericka Dixon, BWB Community Organizer and BWTRC Testifier, August 23, 2016. https://www.goodreads.com/quotes/141138-the-fact-that-we-are-here-and-that-i-speak

5. Melanie Tervalon, MD, MPH, and Jann Murray-Garcia, MD, MPH, Cultural Humility Versus Cultural Competence: A Critical Distinction in Defining Physician Training Outcomes in Multicultural Education. *J Health Care Poor Underserved*. 1998;9(2):117.

6. Katherine A. Yeager, PhD, RN, and Susan Bauer-Wu, PhD, RN, FAAN, Cultural Humility: Essential Foundation for Clinical Researchers. *Appl Nurs Res*. 2013;26(4). doi:10.1016/j.apnr.2013.06.008

7. Z. Kumas-Tan, B. Beagan, C. Loppie, A. MacLeod, and B. Frank, Measures of Cultural Competence: Examining Hidden Assumptions. *Acad Med*. 2007;82(6):548, 551

8. David R. Williams, PhD, MPH, and Ronald Wyatt, MD, MHA, Racial Bias in Health Care and Health: Challenges and Opportunities. *JAMA*. 2015;314(6):556. doi:10.1001/jama.2015.9260

9. Chimamanda Ngozi Adichie, The Danger of a Single Story [TED talk], presented at TEDGlobal 2009, July, Oxford, UK.

10. Yeager and Bauer-Wu, Cultural Humility, p. 4.

11. Yeager and Bauer-Wu, Cultural Humility, p. 4.

12. Lambda Legal, When Health Care Isn't Caring: Transgender and Gender-Nonconforming People Results from Lambda Legal's Health Care Fairness Survey, *Lambda Legal*, New York, 2010, p. 2. https://www.lambdalegal.org/sites/default/files/publications/downloads/whcic-insert_transgender-and-gender-nonconforming-people.pdf

13. Tervalon and Murray-Garcia, Cultural Humility, p. 122.

14. Tervalon and Murray-Garcia, Cultural Humility, p. 122. This list is adapted from the original material.

15. Attributed to a statement Dr. Martin Luther King, Jr., made in Chicago on March 25, 1966, to the second convention of the Medical Committee for Human Rights.

16. Melanie Tervalon, Cultural Humility Training of Trainers, 2015. Summary of Tervalon and Murray-Garcia's Cultural Humility article—prepared for use in a series of training sessions for family partners and clinicians hosted by Every Child Counts Programs, years 2013, 2014, 2015, Alameda County, California.

17. Jack Kornfield, Right Understanding. October 28, 2016. https://jackkornfield.com/right-understanding/

Taking Care of Others and Ourselves: Methods of Humanistic Patient Care and a Guide to Clinician Self-Care

The Essence of Healing

The practice of medicine
Is not what it was
In my grandfather's time.

I remember him telling me
Of weeks that went by
When he would be paid
Only in chickens
Or only in potatoes;

Of treating the families
Of striking miners
In Montrose or Telluride
Who could not pay at all;
Of delivering babies
(A total of twenty)
For a tribe of dirt farmers
Who paid one new-laid egg
Of a cup of springwater;

After sweating a breech birth
And twins at that,
At five in the morning
It was mighty good water.

When fifty years later,
He came back to the mountains
Middle-aged babies
Ran up the street
Crying Doc! Doc! eyes streaming,
Tried to kiss old hands.

No, the practice of medicine
Is not what it was,
But it has its moments:

That morning in surgery
I regained consciousness
A little too early
And found the doctor
Kissing my hand,
Whispering, whispering
It's all right, darling
You're going to live.

—Carolyn Kizer, *Medicine*[i]

Our patients will not remember the sage advice we give them. The confusing medical terms we use will fade into obscurity, and medications we prescribe will be forgotten. All the brilliant interventions we so proudly bestow on them will one day be lost. What they will remember is the kindness, care, and love we give them during the most vulnerable moments of their lives. The relationship between you and your patient is what forges the bond that carries you both through the storms of illness and into the calm seas of healing. This relationship is the essence of the commitment we make when we enter the healing profession. Yet all too often our interactions have become swift, expedient, and impersonal in a fast-food, drive-through healthcare system that is willing to sacrifice our capacity to form a caring relationship in order to save time and money. We can't return to medicine being what it was in Carolyn Kizer's grandpa's time, when an egg or a cup of water was enough, but we can restore the values of compassion and empathy that create meaningful, healing relationships in cancer survivorship.

Medical training and even the more evidence-based psychological schools of thought have moved away from emotional contact into more mechanized, behavioral methods of treatment. Some clinicians are actually instructed not to feel emotion or, if they do, not to show how they feel when they are with their patients. In a written interview on July 18, 2016, Meridithe Mendelsohn, PhD, Program Manager for Cancer Survivorship, told me: "Cancer centers are checking a box and not patient-focused." I believe that this lack of authentic connection is at the heart of the loss of meaning and lagging inspiration that is experienced by many clinicians. When you are trained only to be a technician, you lose the connection both with your patients and, very significantly, with yourself. Meaningful work fades into rote tasks performed *on* others rather than creating a collaborative relationship *with* one another. An authentic relationship reminds us that we can become midwives of the soul when we connect with our patients where they are and nourish both them and ourselves as human beings committed to health and healing. Together in this powerful place of presence with one another, we co-create a healing relationship.

There is, however, substantial evidence that there are significant benefits to training cancer healthcare providers to improve their communication skills: it increases their confidence in responding to emotional cues, managing patient anger and crying, and eliciting patient's emotional concerns—a deeper awareness of the importance of psychosocial issues in routine care.

—Amy E. Lowery, PhD, and Jimmie Holland, MD,
Community Oncology[2]

The Importance of Creating a Healing Relationship

Why is the relationship so crucial to healing? In his book, *Attachment in Psychotherapy*, David Wallin, PhD, quoted the British psychoanalyst John Bowlby: "In a world according to Bowlby, our lives from the cradle to the grave revolve around intimate attachments."[3] We are not meant to live in isolation, and those individuals who are left to face illness without support fare far worse than those with solid support systems. Even the brief intimate interactions that are possible in busy schedules are significant in the satisfaction of our patients and the benefit of our lives as clinicians. The story that follows is a beautiful illustration of the difference that humanistic care can provide.

A young person I see in my psychotherapy practice who is living with a poor cancer prognosis told me numerous stories about stressful interactions with her oncologist. She described lengthy wait times for scan results, insensitive comments about her condition and her concerns, and frightening words spoken in haste.

In many of our sessions together, we discussed her capacity to advocate for herself and her right to be treated in a humanistic way that would help her to get her needs met. With my support, she moved forward and asserted her desire to change oncologists, and with time and tenacity, she transferred to another one. Nervous for her intake interview with the new doctor, she expected a familiar judgment about her treatment history as it involved a choice to halt a treatment that had seriously impacted her quality of life. Instead, she was greeted with an encouraging and compassionate response from the new oncologist, who congratulated her for completing as much of the treatment as she had. This new doctor asked what she needed, what she found helpful and not helpful. She explained to her new doctor that the long waits for results were extremely distressing to her, and he allayed her concerns by telling her she would be provided results on the same day that she was tested. This agreement was successfully met with each following scan and visit. What I witnessed here was the difference in the mood of my client—her sense of renewed hope and gratitude for the care of the oncologist and the smile on her face that told the story better than any words.

Because people remember and value the quality of their relationships, it is important that we commit to learning how to be present in relationship with another human being. While an authentic person-centered relationship does not replace a high standard for medical care, it does enhance the quality of integrated care. We all suffer from a sinking feeling of disconnection in our clinical work when objectivity and detachment are prized over empathy and presence. We experience a restored sense of meaning when we reach a hand out to someone who is in need of our help. After all, this is one of the main reasons many of us became clinicians in the first place.

Psychological education and training are largely missing in most medical programs, both prior to and after licensure, stranding clinicians in a place where they have no tools for dealing with the emotional aspects of illness. How can we expect to bring emotional intelligence to our work if we have not been given the training? How do we include ongoing experiential education and guidance for those skills that involve hands-on learning? Because what is true is that we can't be with others when we have not worked with our own emotional intelligence, accepted our own need for guidance, or asked for help when we needed it. These personal aspects of our education complement our professional training, and both are essential to the practice of integrated healthcare. There is a great need to shift the negative attitudes in the healthcare field toward a more personal relationship style with our patients, which involves providing needed tools for clinicians and giving permission for clinicians to meet their own relational needs.

When I asked (via email, 2016) retired breast surgeon Dr. Jon Greif about the task of attending to the emotional distress of patients, he told me that "some patients do get very emotionally distressed, and dealing with it can be stressful for providers. Some tools to share would be helpful."

I believe that we as physicians need to talk to our cancer survivors about the unique struggles of survivorship. Oncologists need to focus on preparing breast cancer patients for survivorship. That is, they must address the loss experienced by survivors when active treatment is over and they are sent away from a very intense environment. They must help survivors understand the impact of fear and uncertainty on their lives and what might help them reduce these stressors.

—Elizabeth D. McKinley, MD, MPH, "Under Toad Days"[4]

An authentic relationship is built on open and clear communication and an interest in understanding the person with whom you are interacting. This level of connection happens within the relationship itself and is less about the content of the conversation than the shared contact that's experienced by both clinician and patient. The powerful influence of personal experience is the most important place of learning person-centered care. A strong relational capacity is experiential by nature and cannot be fully learned from tools such as worksheets, books, or videos. These are the training tools that give us a structure to work with, but it is important to acknowledge they do not replace the experience of being in a relationship with another person.

Opportunities and ongoing support for personal and interpersonal learning that integrate experiential development with competent knowledge of clinical skills are essential to the clinician's capacity for meaningful clinical work. Relationship skills need to be fostered in a humanistic curriculum that provides creative, supportive, and collaborative learning environments that give clinicians the opportunity to develop their personal leadership skills, their emotional intelligence and their capacity to create authentic human connections.

The Essential Elements of a Healing Relationship

When you are working with a patient, their health status is always the top priority. You do everything in your knowledge to give them the proper medical treatment. After everything is medically attended to, then it is time to heal the person— the individual—by showing empathy, compassion, and an understanding of what he or she is going through.

—Brian Boyle, patient, A Patient's Advice on How to Improve the Health Care Experience[5]

Here, we review the essential interpersonal capacities that clinicians need in order to have healing relationships with their patients: empathy, compassion, kindness, trust, being, authenticity, humor, patience, and personal and professional boundaries. Sometimes referred to as "soft skills," these skills are often dismissed because, unlike technical skills, they are not easily measurable. However, they are not measurable precisely because they call on a true presence of mutual openness to another human being that is not easily quantified. It does, however, require full participation in the areas of reflective and relational understanding, personal development, and honest self-evaluation.

In my education as a depth psychotherapist, we were constantly reminded that the essence of an authentic relationship revolved around the alliance between the clinician and the patient. We were taught that we must first concentrate on forming this alliance, and that only once this connection was well formed could we engage with our patients in direct and meaningful conversations. By forming an alliance with our patients, we create a partnership that allows for a shared experience of empathic connection. When our patients experience this emotional alliance, or empathic rapport, they feel cared for and understood. For clinicians, the experience of this emotional connection with patients feels fulfilling and meaningful, reminding us of why we decided to enter into the healing profession in the first place.

When we create an alliance between ourselves and our patients, we form a partnership that is beneficial to both parties, all the while acknowledging how much we can learn from one another. A clinical relationship that is fostered as a partnership is effective for patients in that they feel joined by their practitioner in both their treatment and survivorship care, which helps them feel less alone as they move forward in their lives. This gives patients a sense of empowerment and guides them in their own resilience, self-efficacy, and willingness to take action on behalf of their own healing. We are stronger when we feel like someone is walking alongside us, when they have our back.

For clinicians who are feeling disconnected and isolated from human interaction, a partnered relationship restores a sense of collaboration. An authentic alliance also allows for the humanity of the clinician, a visibility that says, "I am human, too." In my research, I came on a 2004 interview in *The Morning News* in which Rafael Campo, MD, known for his compassionate and humanistic work in medicine, said: "My colleagues come up to me all the time and say to me, 'How can you be so visible to your patients?' My response to that when it is a party full of doctors: 'I think it is so important a part of my attempt to align myself as a therapeutic ally with my patients to really reveal myself [to be] just as human as they are.'"[6] It's striking to note that this interview took place over a decade ago, showing that the struggles to bring humanistic values into healthcare are still occurring today.

Empathy

Empathy is defined as the ability to sense other people's emotions, coupled with the ability to imagine what someone else might be thinking or feeling. Sensitive individuals are often empathic because they're more naturally tuned in to others. And yet, this is an emotional skill that can be learned and developed through self-reflection, practice, interaction, and personal feedback. Having empathy for our patients demands that we be present with them, be curious about them, ask questions, and then listen to their replies. We can learn a great deal about our patients simply by sitting with them and listening to their concerns. We would do well to spend time in the rich territory of the human heart as a path to discovering the roots of deep compassion for others.

Clinical empathy was once dismissively known as "good bedside manner" and traditionally regarded as far less important than technical acumen.

But a spate of studies in the past decade has found that it is no mere frill. Increasingly, empathy is considered essential to establishing trust, the foundation of a good doctor-patient relationship.

—Sandra G. Goodman, "How to Teach Doctors Empathy"[7]

Compassion

Cancer is no longer a death sentence as science, technology, and growing knowledge based on research have given many people who've been diagnosed with cancer an opportunity to survive. More information on cancer prevention, sophisticated treatments, and the use of diagnostic tools that allow for early detection have saved millions of lives. Yet compassion has probably been the quality that has deeply healed more people in their journey of illness than any medical intervention. When we are compassionate with our patients, they feel held in ways that support their courageous battles with pain, illness, and hardship.

The practice of compassion is challenging in that it takes us to the edge of our comfort zone with people and in situations that are fraught with the difficulties of time and personal energy. Pema Chodrun wrote: "When we set out to support other human beings, when we go so far as to stand in their shoes, when we aspire to never close down to anyone, we quickly find ourselves in the uncomfortable territory of 'life not on my terms.'"[8] She also suggested a practice of opening our door to everyone, gradually and with an awareness of our own comfort and discomfort, giving ourselves permission to open and close the door as needed. Caring for another human being with an open mind and heart is a continual practice of learning compassion in the moments with our patients. Bringing our compassion into our clinical relationships is constantly challenged by time constraints, overloaded schedules, exhaustion, and personal difficulties; at the same time, remaining open to others gives us a renewed sense of meaning.

Compassion is our deepest nature. It arises from our interconnections with all things.

—Jack Kornfield, *The Wise Heart*[9]

Kindness

No act of kindness, no matter how small, is ever wasted.

—Aesop

Kindness is a state of mind, a way of choosing how to be in the world that makes a profound difference. In healthcare, when we come from a place of kindness in our interactions with our patients, their partners, and their family members, we let them know that we care about them as a whole human being, not just another clinical case with a number attached. Like empathy, kindness requires no additional time, as it is a felt sense from another person that conveys warmth and concern. A touch, a kind word, and taking a moment to listen are all very significant to the experience of our patients during times of heightened fear and chaos. Our kind and engaged presence is instrumental to the enhancement of the experience of our patients and their supporters.

A recent study by Wakefield Research for Dignity Health confirmed that delivering care with kindness matters and reported that

Eighty-seven percent of Americans feel that kind treatment by a physician is more important than other key considerations in choosing a healthcare provider, including average wait time before appointments, distance from home and the cost of care. These feelings are so powerful that they help patients to decide where to seek treatment and how much they are willing to pay for it. The Wakefield survey revealed that nearly three-fourths of respondents would be willing to pay more to visit healthcare providers who emphasized kindness in their treatment approach. In addition, nearly 88 percent are willing to travel farther to receive kinder care.[10]

A kind approach can also extend into our relationships with our colleagues. Our place of work, regardless of setting, will only benefit from all of us treating one another with respect and kindness. This type of collaboration creates a ripple effect from one another to our patients, to their support systems, and into the world. Integrated care that does not exclude the needs of the clinicians builds a kinder, more inclusive workplace.

Trust

To me the ideal doctor would be a man endowed with profound knowledge of life and of the soul, intuitively divining any suffering or disorder of whatever kind, and restoring peace by his mere presence.

—Henri-Frederic Amiel, *The Journal Intime of Henri-Frederic Amiel*[11]

Trust happens in relationships with our patients when we meet them where they are and when we let them know that we care about what matters to them. Rosemary Rowe and Michael Calnan, in their article "Trust Relations in Health Care—The New Agenda," wrote: "The need for interpersonal trust relates to the vulnerability associated with being ill, the information asymmetries arising from the competence and intentions of the practitioner on whom the patient is dependent."[12]

We earn the trust of our patients by coming from a place of transparency that is built on our personal commitment to our professional development as well as our own well-developed, genuine presence and authentic communication with others.

Trust between clinician and patient does not mean blind faith in the words and actions of the clinician. A trusting clinical relationship consists of two or more individuals who trust their own thoughts, feelings, and intuitions and who believe that the other individual in the relationship is honest and has a sincere interest in their welfare. From this foundation, a partnership based on mutual trust and respect is formed. Building trust in a clinical relationship starts with the initial contact and continues to grow throughout the relationship. While it is personal, trust also means that we are professional in our clinical relationships, holding a strong framework that has strong and fluid boundaries, is based on competence, and strives to offer accurate information and quality services to our patients. People respond well to transparency in a relationship as it strips away layers of inauthentic communication and "cuts to the chase."

Being

The process of be-ing is the process of life.

—James F. T. Bugental, *The Search for Authenticity*[13]

Being is another word for the process of awareness or consciousness. Awareness is the doorway to discovering our essential self, our being. Existential thought holds as a basic fact that existence is existence and identifies the significance of existence as the potentiality for being. Then, we travel full circle to the experience of existence as awareness. When we allow ourselves to be present with who we are, we tap into a sense of timelessness that is profoundly freeing.

Sometimes we need to take the time to reflect on who we are and not just stay within the roles we have chosen that define us in certain ways. While being is often a reflective process, it can also move us to action. This type of action is not necessarily about taking care of the tasks on your to-do list, but highlights a deeper personal motivation that includes attention to what really matters to you in your life. Deeper explorations could include creativity, dreams, and intentions that take into account the bigger picture of your life, realizations of what you believe to be important to you.

There will be many times in our clinical relationships when words or actions fall short. A patient can feel joined and comforted in quiet moments of being together in silence.

Authenticity

The quality the relationship needs to have as much as possible is authenticity.

—James F. T. Bugental, *Psychotherapy and Process*[14]

The clinical relationship has the potential to become a partnership of human healing and growth where both people involved bring, to the best of their abilities, a genuine presence to the interactions. Authenticity means that we commit to self-awareness, accept that we have choice, and take responsibility for our decisions. It is our job as clinicians to provide a safe setting for our patients to express themselves and where we can bring ourselves to our work as aware and authentic in our caring for others. Both patient and clinician agree to risk being present in an authentic relationship with one another.

The actualization of being helps us find the courage to live authentically. We communicate and connect from a place within us that is aware, grounded, and aligned with what we are feeling and thinking. Rather than reacting from an outward or surface place, we respond from within ourselves. In my work with clients, I call this moving from in to out. Genuine responsiveness and good choices occur when we come from an authentic inner place.

Patience

The more you know yourself, the more patience you have for what you see in others. You don't have to accept what people do, but understand what leads them to do it.

—Joan Serson Erikson, interview with Daniel Goleman,
New York Times[15]

Learning the art of patience helps you develop the capacity to take things as they come without fighting every frustration, setback, and misunderstanding you may endure in your clinical practice. Being able to roll with things as they happen with a calm and patient attitude is the best remedy for difficult and distressing events and interactions. This stance of harmonious communication with others helps to balance the stresses inherent in your daily work and is an essential aspect of compassion.

When you are patient, you come from a place of personal power within yourself in order to better respond to a troublesome situation or a frustrating personal interaction. Being patient involves relaxing into times of waiting and uncertainty without the need to push forward. You can prevent becoming overwhelmed or irritated and avoid giving up or blaming others. Instead, you remain in a balanced state that aids you in being centered in yourself. Practicing patience will help you relieve your stress and give you the opportunity to make choices about how you respond in demanding moments. You may experience a sense of freedom in meeting things (and people) as they are.

Humor

Doctors said that the test most commonly used to screen for colon cancer doesn't go far enough. They're recommending a procedure that involves photographing the entire colon. I say, don't give CBS an idea for another reality show.

—Bill Maher[16]

A good laugh when you are working with people who are struggling with a scary cancer diagnosis can sometimes give a temporary reprieve from gnawing feelings of sadness, replacing fear with humor. A diagnosis of cancer and its grueling treatments are incredibly stressful. Humor may help to ease the trauma and bring some humanity to the infusion rooms and treatment centers. Humor can lighten the mood during difficult moments, whether you are patient or clinician. Indeed, laughing with our colleagues can cheer us on through our own rough moods and times of exhaustion. Humor connects us in ways that can soften the blows of distress and isolation experienced by patients, clinicians, families, and caregivers.

We work with cancer patients because we have a desire to help them heal and sometimes to simply help them feel better. When used sensitively, we can learn to use humor to help create a healing environment both for our patients and for our colleagues. As clinicians, we need to pay attention to the humor used by our patients and to join them in a little levity when we can. Humor in our clinical work needs to come from the heart, have its roots in a respectful caring, and encourage an empathic understanding with our patients. Humor can be instrumental in creating a relationship of friendliness based on trust and warm interpersonal connection.

Personal and Professional Boundaries

The most important distinction anyone can ever make in their life is between who they are as an individual and their connection with others.

—Anné Linden, *Boundaries in Human Relationships*[17]

Boundaries are essentially about recognizing and honoring personal space. When we follow this simple instruction, we form alliances with our patients that are ethical and empathic. As clinicians, we are responsible for our professional boundaries as well as our personal boundaries and how we take care of ourselves both in our work and in our personal lives. A professional boundary is the frame that both holds and defines what is included or excluded within the clinical relationship. This includes articulating a distinct structure of services being provided, as well as a commitment to professional responsibilities and behaviors that champion the needs of our patients.

Critical areas relevant to establishing ethical clinical boundaries include time, place, space, money, gifts, services, clothing, language, self-disclosure, and physical contact. These are the more obvious, or black-and-white, aspects of professional boundaries. There are, however, large gray areas where boundaries are concerned that aren't as easily "regulated" because they interweave with the personal relationships we may develop with our patients. These areas may include self-disclosure, bending the rules to attend more personally to a patient, showing affection, and other ways of moving beyond the black-and-white frame of the agreed-on relationship in order to create a more humanistic relationship. Walking in this gray territory requires self-awareness, integrity, and attention to power dynamics, as well as transparency. The bottom line remains that all care and interactions be based on the best interests of the patient.

The responsibility of holding a clear, strong, yet fluid boundary in clinical relationships can be challenging. You may find yourself struggling with difficult patients who are pushing and pulling on you for a level of emotional care that you simply cannot provide to them. Your work in cancer survivorship can take a frightening turn at any moment when a patient or family crisis occurs. Then there are those times when your own life is so exhausting or stressful that it's hard to find the strength of heart within yourself to be present. Personal and professional boundaries are not static, but rather constantly changing depending on the circumstances of the day or the issues of the patient. Maintaining your integrity in lieu of these shifting realities can become slippery. Conversations and feedback from colleagues are good reality checks, as is professional consultation to help you continue to understand and work with the boundaries of your clinical relationships.

A cancer diagnosis affects those who are in a relationship with the patient. Partners and families are interrelated with one another, so the effect of cancer on the family affects the health and well-being of all of those involved. Relationships where cancer is present can be at risk for high levels of stress, and these stresses may continue well into the patient's survivorship. Cancer, its treatments, and then the phases of survivorship can cause myriad complex feelings for all concerned. Life changes that were not chosen can be equally overwhelming for partners and families as for patients. Good communication is important in our relationships with both our patients *and* the people who care about them.

How do we support the people who are connected with a cancer patient? My book *Surviving the Storm: A Workbook for Telling Your Cancer Story* (Krauter, 2017) includes a chapter on this group of partners, family members, and friends, with suggestions for them about how to address their own needs when a loved one is struggling with cancer. You may find this section of *Surviving the Storm* helpful in your interactions with partners and families. You might also think about creating a type of distress screening form for partners and families to address their concerns, which can also give you valuable information regarding your patient's situation. These people matter because they provide information about the context and quality of a relationship that affect how the person with cancer responds to his or her disease. This same relational context is known to affect the quality of self-care for partners and family members.

The impact of cancer has been compared to casting a stone into water. The illness creates a ripple that spreads outward and changes daily life as it has been known. Some of these changes can have a long-lasting impact on all of those involved, regardless of outcomes. The needs of partners, family members, and friends of cancer survivors have generally not been acknowledged, and this group has traditionally slipped through the cracks. Identifying their needs and offering support and resources to help them process their experience with cancer is instrumental in survivorship care that is holistic and humanistic.

*He [Oliver Sacks] wrote to vivify each patient's unique experience,
often using their own idiosyncratic speech. He listened not only
with a stethoscope, but a poet's ear.*

—Norman Doidge, "Every Patient Has a Story Worth Hearing"[18]

A poet's ear listens deeply to the world and often translates universal themes about the human condition into words that touch the heart. Perhaps the well-honed craft of the poet is elusive for clinicians, yet the skills of listening, being present, and engaging in compassionate conversations are foundational aspects of a humanistic, healing relationship. This emotional level of care matters to our patients and gives meaning and aliveness to our work as clinicians. It is clear that a good patient experience and clinician satisfaction both matter in cancer survivorship care.

In an article in the *Patient Experience Journal,* Jason Wolf, PhD, wrote: "Clinical outcomes are unquestionably the primary focus in healthcare. This is not simply a healing effort but one that commits to well-being and honors that in some circumstances all that can be done is ensure an individual can live their remaining moments with dignity."[19] The emphasis on end-of-life care is, without a doubt, essential, as is the commitment to well-being and dignity in survivorship care, even if this is at times more complex for the practitioner. Our patients have had the fortune to survive cancer, but they are still left to heal from the trauma they have undergone.

The following workbook sections provide guidance to enhance the human quality of the clinical relationship and offer exercises and worksheets that include how to have healing conversations, pitfalls in our clinical work, and structures for meaningful interview processes with our patients. You may pick and choose the sections that feel pertinent to you depending on your concerns at any given moment. You may also want to spend some reflective time with these questions or prompts when you are looking at the bigger picture of your clinical work and how you want to be in relationships with your patients.

The Essentials of a Healing Relationship in Survivorship Care

Empathy

- How do you feel when you interact with your patients?

_____

_____

_____

_____

- Do you feel present when you are with your patients, or are you distracted or preoccupied? How much do you allow yourself to be present with them?

_____

_____

_____

_____

- What is your comfort level with personal interaction with your patients? How willing are you to stay with conversations that are uncomfortable?

_____

_____

_____

_____

- Do you allow yourself to identify or relate with the experiences, thoughts, and feelings of your patients? If so, how much do you self-disclose?

_____

_____

_____

_____

■ Are you curious about the person you are with, not just the patient you are treating?

_____

_____

_____

_____

■ How do you want to show up as a clinician? How do you bring awareness to your own personal relational style and the kinds of wants, issues, and challenges that you face in your clinical work?

_____

_____

_____

_____

■ How meaningful are your relationships with your patients? Do you feel that your alliance with them is what you would like it to be?

_____

_____

_____

_____

■ How do you experience your humanity in your work? Are you satisfied? Are you content?

_____

_____

_____

_____

■ Do you feel engaged, connected, and alive with the people you work with?

_____

_____

_____

_____

Ways to Develop Empathy

- Start with yourself. Discover, develop, and commit to an ongoing practice of self-reflection that expands your personal empathic stance both toward others and within yourself.
- Listen to the person and bring your attention to your own experience. Notice your own feelings, thoughts, and body sensations as a way to join the person, understand their experience, and build a stronger relationship.
- Make eye contact.
- Pay attention to the tone of your voice and your body posture. Notice the vocal tone and body posture of your patient.
- Look through the eyes of a cancer patient. Spend some time in the infusion chair, or lay down in a magnetic resonance imaging machine or on a radiology table. Imagine the moment of getting a cancer diagnosis and see what you experience.
- Practice cultural humility by being aware of biases and assumptions about another person's experience. Align with them by asking about their background, their beliefs, their identity.
- Recognize the signs of empathic breakdown and seek help to understand the issues to better restore affinity, responsiveness, and warmth.

Compassion

- Are you compassionate with yourself? In what ways do you practice bringing compassion for yourself into your professional and personal life?

_____

_____

_____

_____

- Are you harder on yourself than on others?

_____

_____

_____

_____

- When you're having a difficult time, do you feel inadequate? Are you judgmental of yourself and others in stressful, frustrating situations?

_____

_____

_____

_____

- Is it okay to be human in your clinical work?

_____

_____

_____

_____

- How do you cope with the challenges of bringing compassion into your clinical relationships considering time constraints, overloaded schedules, and exhaustion? How do these issues affect your capacity to remain open to others?

_____

_____

_____

_____

- Do you feel that you bring an open heart and a spacious mind to your relationships? What do you notice when your heart is shut and your mind is closed?

_____

_____

_____

_____

- When is it hard for you to have compassion for yourself? What do you understand about this difficulty?

_____

_____

- When is it hard for you to have compassion for others? For example, are there certain situations, or specific personality types, that are difficult for you to deal with? How do you understand the places inside of you that struggle with feeling compassionate toward others?

_____

_____

_____

_____

- How do you understand and relate to unconditional positive regard for another human being? What are your strengths? What are your challenges?

_____

_____

_____

_____

Ways to Develop Compassion

- Find time each morning to reflect on bringing a compassionate attitude to your day. This may take the form of meditation, contemplation, affirmation, or whatever form that speaks to you and helps you to have an open heart with yourself and with others.
- In the evening, give yourself a few moments to reflect on your day. Focus on the interactions with patients and colleagues and bring your attention to how you feel as you review your day. Be open and kind with yourself.
- Notice your judgments and do the best you can to suspend them and focus on being present with your patient.
- Find a personal statement to say silently within yourself that conveys your compassionate understanding. For example, "This person is in pain, and I wish an end to suffering for them."

- When you have difficult or frustrating interactions, try to remember the stress the patient is enduring, their background, and the physical and emotional pain they are in. By not personalizing their reactions, you can move from reaction into a responsive place.
- Develop self-compassion by thinking of your own difficulties and then observing your thoughts and feelings. Be aware of anger, self-recrimination, fear, and all the ways that you turn away from having a loving attitude toward yourself. Notice what happens by shifting your thoughts to engage a warm, supportive, and accepting attitude.
- Have a short statement that you carry within yourself throughout the day that opens your heart and your mind and reminds you of the simple, powerful practice of compassion. For example, "May all beings everywhere be safe, be happy, be free of suffering" or "May I be peaceful and happy, at ease in my body and my mind."

Kindness

- What does being kind mean to you?

_____

_____

_____

_____

- Do you feel like you consciously choose to be kind?

_____

_____

_____

_____

- Do you give yourself the same kindness you give to others? Reflect on this and see what emerges for you.

_____

_____

_____

_____

- How do you let your patients know that you care about them?

_____

_____

_____

_____

- Do you feel comfortable touching your patient as a way to alleviate their suffering or cheer them up?

_____

_____

_____

_____

- How much do you believe that you don't have the time to be in your interactions with your patients? How does this affect you?

_____

_____

_____

_____

- In what ways do you access your inner resources so that you can act with kindness toward others?

_____

_____

_____

_____

- How are you generous with yourself when you are having a difficult time?

_____

_____

_____

_____

Ways to Develop Kindness

- Pause before you speak in order to be thoughtful in your words and actions.
- Find something positive to say about the person you are with.
- Think of small gestures or comforts that are kind and supportive.
- Let the person you are with know that you care about them.
- Take the time to listen, even if you have heard the story before.
- Consider making contact with a human touch that is appropriate.
- Express gratitude to and for others.
- Practice being generous with others and yourself.

Trust

- Describe how you build interpersonal trust with your patients.

_____

_____

_____

_____

- Are you comfortable with your own vulnerability when you are with your patients?

_____

_____

_____

_____

- How much do you allow yourself to be transparent with your patients?

_____

_____

_____

_____

- In what ways do you assure your patients of your competence, letting them know that they are "in good hands"?

_____

_____

_____

_____

- Do you feel satisfied with your ongoing process of personal and professional development? Would you like to change the level of commitment to your own competence?

_____

_____

_____

_____

- How comfortable are you with being direct with your patients? Do you feel okay about owning what you don't know or understand?

_____

_____

_____

_____

- What does an honest, trustworthy clinical relationship mean to you? What does it feel like?

_____

_____

_____

_____

Ways to Develop Trust

- Start by making a personal connection.
- Make eye contact.

- Prepare for the appointment (e.g., review the chart, notes, records).
- Find a common language with your patient (e.g., no medical jargon).
- Give your patient your full attention.
- Acknowledge when you are late, haven't returned messages, or anything that has disrupted the trust in the relationship.
- Listen to your patient and engage them in the interaction with you.

Being

- How are you present in your conversations with your patients?

_____

_____

_____

_____

- Do you feel comfortable with stillness, being in silence, attending to nonverbal cues?

_____

_____

_____

_____

- Are you aware of when you need to listen? What type of reflection or inner awareness helps you with the skill of listening?

_____

_____

_____

_____

- What's it like for you to sit with uncertainty?

_____

_____

_____

_____

How do you work with the existential reality of "existence is existence," meaning that sometimes we must face life as it is and let go of the illusion of control?

_____

_____

_____

_____

How comfortable are you with moving out of your prescribed clinical role and letting go of tasks that involve something to do, giving advice, or other action-oriented activities?

_____

_____

_____

_____

Do you give yourself the time and space for personal reflection? How do you tap into your own field of being in order to discover and affirm what matters to you?

_____

_____

_____

_____

Ways to Develop Being

- Check in regularly with yourself to see where you are in the moment.
- Pay attention to body sensations.
- Bring awareness to your breath.
- Slow down.
- Notice when you are in the future or in the past rather than the present moment.
- Give yourself the space to stretch and move your body.
- Practice letting go of the need to do or fix something.
- Explore and develop a contemplative practice.

Authenticity

- Do you feel that you are as fully aware as you can be? As aware as you want to be?

_____

_____

_____

_____

- What do you believe about your capacity for choice in your work? In your life?

_____

_____

_____

_____

- Do you experience a sense of belonging in your life? Describe this experience. Describe what it is like if the experience of belonging is a challenge for you.

_____

_____

_____

_____

- Do you think you are working in creative, meaningful ways that are congruent to who you are? Is this sometimes a struggle for you?

_____

_____

_____

_____

- Do you feel a sense of harmony and connection within yourself as well as in the work that you do? Reflect on this.

_____

_____

_____

_____

▪ Do you feel that you can be yourself in your interactions with your patients? What about in your interactions with colleagues?

_____

_____

_____

_____

▪ Do you feel the freedom to be truly open? Reflect and comment on your experience.

_____

_____

_____

_____

Ways to Develop Authenticity

▪ Choose and commit to an ongoing practice of self-awareness.
▪ Connect with your capacity to make choices.
▪ Explore and become familiar with your own genuine presence.
▪ Find your courage.
▪ Risk showing up as who you are.
▪ Seek genuine connections with both patients and colleagues.
▪ Explore and discover what personal transparency means to you.

Patience

▪ What's it like for you to accept people as they are?

_____

_____

_____

_____

- How do you work with patience as a way to accept people and situations?

_____

_____

_____

_____

- How do you recognize when you are impatient? What are the thoughts, feelings, physical sensations you experience that let you know you're being impatient?

_____

_____

_____

_____

- How do you react to delays, frustrating interactions, and trouble-some situations? What happens inside you during these moments?

_____

_____

_____

_____

- How do you let yourself relax?

_____

_____

_____

_____

- How does an experience of feeling overwhelmed affect your ability to be patient?

_____

_____

_____

_____

How do you work with the ability to contain your emotional reactions or impulses so that you can proceed calmly when faced with difficulties?

_____

_____

_____

_____

Ways to Develop Patience

- Choose and develop a personal relaxation practice.
- Meet people and situations as they are.
- Slow down and take a breath.
- Give yourself a break both internally and externally.
- Practice thinking before speaking.
- Respond rather than react.
- Learn to be patient with yourself.

Humor

Do you use humor as a way to connect with your patients? How?

_____

_____

_____

_____

Do you use humor to connect with your colleagues? How?

_____

_____

_____

_____

- What have you learned about and from your patients by engaging in a humorous interaction?

_____

_____

_____

_____

- Are you comfortable with using humor in your interactions with patients? If not, would you like to feel more comfortable with humor?

_____

_____

_____

_____

- How do you assess whether the use of humor is appropriate?

_____

_____

_____

_____

- Do you believe laughter is beneficial to a healing environment? Why or why not?

_____

_____

_____

_____

- Can you laugh at yourself in a nonpejorative manner?

_____

_____

_____

_____

Ways to Develop Humor

- Learn to laugh at yourself.
- Spend time with playful people.
- Find short funny videos to watch on your phone.
- Share a funny story or joke.
- Connect with the spontaneous and silly child within you.
- Spend time with children.
- Share laughter with your colleagues.

Personal and Professional Boundaries

- Do you feel that you have a clear understanding of your professional boundaries as they relate to the basic framework of the work you are doing (e.g., fees, appointment schedules, agreed-on services)?

_____

_____

_____

_____

- How comfortable are you with making choices that may best serve your patient when it means moving beyond the prescribed framework?

_____

_____

_____

_____

- In what ways do you create a safe environment for your patients?

_____

_____

_____

_____

- What helps you to decide how you self-disclose and what you share personally with your patients? With your colleagues?

_____

_____

_____

_____

- How do you handle physical contact or touch with your patients?

_____

_____

_____

_____

- Describe what an attitude of caring contact looks and feels like to you.

_____

_____

_____

_____

- How do you bring your awareness to when you are either overinvolved or underinvolved with your patients?

_____

_____

_____

_____

- Do you seek regular consultation? Describe this process and think about what is helpful to you.

_____

_____

_____

_____

Ways to Develop Boundaries

- Continue your education on clinical standards and ethics in your field.
- Seek ongoing consultation especially when you feel overwhelmed in your work.
- Self-knowledge is the basis for clarity in terms of your own boundaries. Commit to an ongoing practice of self-knowledge so that you continue to build personal awareness. Focus your attention and intention on the best interests of the patient.
- Always honor and respect personal space.
- Develop a capacity for flexible boundaries.
- Commit to a practice of self-care that helps you discover and establish personal boundaries that will enhance the quality of your clinical work.

The Clinical Interview

A healing relationship is formed in the connection between the clinician and the patient during the clinical interview. While there may not always be the luxury of the time that is afforded in a more traditional psychological interview, it is still essential that, regardless of time, an empathic kinship is formed. Clinicians often fear that opening Pandora's box of emotion and trauma will overwhelm both the patient and themselves, yet, in truth, quite the opposite is true. In reality, it is less about the available amount of time that is practical and possible than it is about an authentic concern and curiosity expressed by the clinician that makes the difference.

It takes education, training, and practical experience to do a skillful clinical interview. However, what is most important is the genuine concern of the clinician for their patient. A sensitive and caring attitude will always be remembered and trusted regardless of whatever outer circumstances are present. Keep in mind that you are talking with people who are dealing with frightening and confusing issues and bring a thoughtful attitude to your conversation. Always remember that your words and actions have impact.

He said it doesn't look good
he said it looks bad in fact real bad
he said I counted thirty-two of them on one lung before
I quit counting them
I said I'm glad I wouldn't want to know
about any more being there than that
he said are you a religious man do you kneel down
in forest groves and let yourself ask for help
when you come to a waterfall
mist blowing against your face and arms
do you stop and ask for understanding at those moments
I said not yet but I intend to start today
he said I'm real sorry he said
I wish I had some other kind of news to give you
I said Amen and he said something else
I didn't catch and not knowing what else to do
and not wanting him to have to repeat it
and me to have to fully digest it
I just looked at him
for a minute and he looked back it was then
I jumped up and shook hands with this man who'd just given me
something no one else on earth had ever given me
I may have even thanked him habit being so strong

—Raymond Carver, "What the Doctor Said"[20]

The Initial Interview

The first step in creating a healing relationship is forming an alliance with your patient. There is nothing more essential than building the patient–clinician alliance, and nothing should be allowed to get in the way of it. A powerful patient–clinician alliance is formed when forces are joined that energize and support the long, difficult, and frequently painful work of counseling someone through a cancer diagnosis and treatment and then into survivorship. The process of building an alliance must start with the initial contact made in the first interview.

Introduce yourself to the patient and engage them in conversation. A few minutes of personal contact makes an enormous difference, as it establishes a feeling of trust that you are, indeed, interested and concerned about the patient as a person and the patient is not just another case number in your clinical practice. Open a dialogue that allows room for the patient to introduce themselves to you, as this will not only build rapport, but also provide you with valuable information about them. Remember that your patient is likely to be frightened or overwhelmed and may need support in understanding what they are facing or have faced. Give the patient time to talk while you listen and then proceed with your own necessary agenda. Your empathic and open demeanor will allow an intimate feeling in what is all too often a sterile and soulless atmosphere.

Suggestions for a Successful First Interview

- Prepare for the meeting by reviewing your notes.
- Know the patient's name and use it in conversation.
- Silence beepers, turn off phones, close the door to the interview room.
- Let the patient begin with their concerns.
- Don't interrupt.
- Practice active listening.
- Check in with the patient to be sure you have understood them.
- Observe the nonverbal cues that the patient communicates.
- Be sensitive to the nonverbal messages that you are conveying.
- Be aware of how you respond to cultural issues.
- Check back in with the patient prior to ending the interview.
- End the interview by clarifying the next steps and make the next appointment.

The Ongoing Relationship

It is essential for you to consider what your choices are in terms of continuity with your patients when they finish active treatment and enter into survivorship. The end of treatment and the beginning of the initial phase of survivorship is another time of concern and uncertainty for cancer patients, their partners, and their families. It's important to recognize this transition, acknowledge that your relationship with them will change, take the time to ask about their needs as they embark on the next leg of their experience with cancer, and provide referrals and resources for their unique needs and concerns.

The level of contact you have had with your patient will likely diminish as they move forward into their life. You may see them every couple of months for a while, then 6 months, then once a year. Survivors can feel lost and even abandoned during this transition because you are no longer monitoring them so closely, which makes it an excellent time to help them negotiate their entry into survivorship. For a significant period of time, you have been a lifeline in their experience with a cancer diagnosis, the person they turned to for information, for guidance, for reassurance. All of us need to consider the fact that we have been far more important to our patients than they have been to us. This is not because of a lack of caring; it simply takes into account the need for a heightened sensitivity in recognizing our importance to each single patient we treat.

Your patients may want to continue to talk with you or see you with more regularity due to the bond that was created throughout the storms of their cancer experience. Our commitment to the ongoing care of our patients is an essential aspect of our professional ethics as clinicians; therefore, we are responsible for providing referrals and resources for them. Keep a working list of trusted referrals and meet with those individuals so you can get a sense of providing a good fit for your patients. Making this list of local professionals, online resources, survivor groups, and workshops available to give to your patients and their families will help them feel held and cared for as they navigate the waters of survivorship. In the end, as clinicians, we may at times be the ones to hold the hope, strength, and faith in our patients until they are strong enough to do it for themselves. Our belief in the power of growth and healing may be the single most significant gift we can give to our patients as they face forward and walk into their new life as a cancer survivor.

Suggestions on Structuring Ongoing Relationships

- Decide how you want to handle your ongoing relationships with patients.
- Acknowledge the reality that you will have less contact with them.
- Realize and pay attention to the bond your patient feels with you.
- Speak to the journey that you have traveled together.
- Ask your patient about their emotional needs now that they have finished cancer treatment.

- Be sure to listen and and ask questions about the concerns that they bring up during your conversation with them.
- Discuss in detail their feelings, thoughts, and experience of their quality of life.
- Provide referrals and resources to qualified clinicians for the emotional healing of the trauma of cancer.

Ways of Supporting the Healing Relationship

- Seek ongoing personal and professional consultation to support yourself in your work.
- Keep the focus of your clinical work on healing at all levels: physical, emotional, intellectual, and spiritual.
- Create alliances with psychology programs, social work programs, and clinicians in a private practice setting to support your work with your patients.
- Gain familiarity of cancer survivorship resources both in your local area and with valid online sites that help cancer survivors.
- Create and use a referral system to psychotherapists, support groups, survivorship workshops and conferences.
- Make a commitment to a caring, empathic connection the foundation of your clinical work with patients.
- Participate in ongoing professional development, such as classes, workshops, educational experiences.
- Establish continuing practices that support your own growth and development as a human being.
- Remember to value and find opportunities that involve experiential learning with others.

All of these tools and suggestions encourage us to be fully present within ourselves and others. It is in the present moment that we join together as human beings regardless of what we do or where we are from. This is the essence of the healing relationship and its power to heal not only our patients but also ourselves.

> *Be fully present*
> *Feel your heart*
> *And engage in the next moment without an agenda*
>
> —Pema Chodron, *Living Beautifully with Uncertainty and Change* [21]

Notes

1. Carolyn Kizer, Medicine, in *Yin*. Copyright © 1984 by Carolyn Kizer. Reprinted with the permission of The Permissions Company, Inc., on behalf of BOA Editions, Ltd., www.boaeditions.org.

2. Amy E. Lowery, PhD, and Jimmie Holland, MD, Screening Cancer Patients for Distress and Guidelines for Routine Implementation [Review]. *J Community Support Oncol.* 2011 Nov 1. https://www.mdedge.com/jcso/article/47002/practice-management/screening-cancer-patients-distress-guidelines-routine?channel=270.

3. David J. Wallin, PhD, *Attachment in Psychotherapy*, Guilford Press, New York, 2017.

4. Elizabeth D. McKinley, MD, MPH, Under Toad Days: Surviving the Uncertainty of Cancer Recurrence. *Ann Intern Med.* 2000;133(6):480.

5. Brian Boyle, patient, A Patient's Advice on How to Improve the Health Care Experience. KevinMD.com. https://www.kevinmd.com/blog/2016/11/patients-advice-improve-health-care-experience.html. Published November 7, 2016. Excerpt from *The Patient Experience* by Brian Boyle is reprinted with the permission of Skyhorse Publishing, Inc.

6. Robert Birnbaum, Rafael Campo. *The Morning News*. https://themorningnews.org/article/birnbaum-v.-rafael-campo. January 29, 2004, p. 7.

7. Sandra G. Goodman, How to Teach Doctors Empathy. *The Atlantic*, March 15, 2015, p. 2.

8. Pema Chodrun, *Living Beautifully with Uncertainty and Change*, Shambhala, Boston, 2012, p. 65.

9. Jack Kornfield, *The Wise Heart: A Guide to the Universal Teachings of Buddhist Psychology*, Bantam Dell, Division of Random House, New York, 2008, p. 23.

10. Recent study by Wakefield Research for Dignity Health, press release from Dignity Health, November 13, 2013, p. 1.

11. Henri-Frederic Amiel, *The Journal Intime of Henri-Frederic Amiel*, August 22, 1883, translated by Mrs. Mary Humphrey Ward (1889), Burton, New York, 1889, Vol. 2, p. 15.

12. Rosemary Rowe and Michael Calnan, Trust Relations in Health Care—The New Agenda. *Eur J Public Health.* 2006;16(1):4. http://eurpub.oxfordjournals.org/content/16/1/4.

13. James F. T. Bugental, *Psychotherapy and Process: The Fundamentals of an Existential-Humanistic Approach*, Addison-Wesley, Boston, 1978, p. 104.

14. Bugental, *Psychotherapy and Process*, p. 104.

15. Joan Serson Erikson, interview with Daniel Goleman. *New York Times*, June 14, 1988. http://www.nytimes.com/books/99/08/22/specials/erikson-old.html.

16. Bill Maher, in Humorous Cancer Quotes and Sayings. n.d. Cancer Is Not Funny website. http://www.cancerisnotfunny.com/quotes.html.

17. Anné Linden, *Boundaries in Human Relationships: How to Be Separate and Connected*, Crown House, Bancyfelin, Wales, 2008. https://www.goodreads.com/work/quotes/2923460-boundaries-in-human-relationships-how-to-be-separate-and-connected.

18. Norman Doidge, Every Patient Has a Story Worth Hearing [Blog]. *Stanford Medicine 25*. https://stanford25blog.stanford.edu/2016/03/every-patient-has-a-story-worth-hearing/. Published March 22, 2016.

19. Jason Wolf, PhD, Patient Experience: Driving Outcomes at the Heart of Healthcare. *Patient Experience J*. 2016;3(1), p. 2.

20. Raymond Carver, What the Doctor Said, in *All of Us: Collected Poems*, Harvill Press, London, 1996. © Harvill Press, 1996, p. 113.

21. Chodron, *Living Beautifully*, p. 21.

CHAPTER 6 — Surviving Our Work

Self-Care, Burnout, and Finding Meaning

For whole days will move in the direction of rain
For you will cry and there will be no one to talk to
    or no one but yourself
For you will be lonely
For you will be alone
For there is a difference
For there is no seriousness like joy
For there is no joy like seriousness
For the days will run together in gallops and the years
    go by as fast as the speed of thought
    which is faster than the speed of light
    or Superman
    or Superwoman
    For you will not be Superman
    For you will not be Superwoman

—John Stone, "Gaudeamust Igitur"[1]

The question: "How do you take care of yourself?" gives most of us pause. How do we answer that often complicated question with a genuine response? We might feel uncomfortable speaking out loud about the very real struggles we face as we attempt that elusive life–work balance we are all constantly striving to create. We might even wonder what we're really talking about when the theme of self-care is mentioned. When is the last time you spent time reflecting on your own needs or acknowledging the thoughts and feelings within you that are demanding attention? Self-care is not just taking the occasional spa day but an ongoing commitment coming from your inner world that has an essential impact on the life you choose to live.

You take care of others. You endeavor to take care of yourself. Within a complex web of other clinicians, you are left to cope with your own pain, stress, and struggles with burnout quietly, often feeling alone in a system that is overloaded and underfunded. You may face ancient, worn-out beliefs telling you that it's selfish to think of your own needs and wants as a clinician. There is an unspoken rule that those of us who work in the healing profession should be selfless and, at times, self-sacrificing. This level of disconnection from the authentic self creates failure to listen to ourselves, which can often lead to a crushing feeling of loneliness. Integrative care paying attention to the whole person is becoming more of a focus in the care of patients. Why not for the clinicians, too?

Self-care is an ongoing commitment to your own well-being not only in the work that you do but also in other areas of your life. Fundamentally, the elusive pursuit of life–work balance rests in the always-shifting arena of giving attention to who you are, where you are, and what you need. You slide into a disconnected and dispirited place when you lose track of intentions that include your continual exploration, growth, and renewal. Burnout is a state of being that is littered with forgotten priorities, leaving you feeling disengaged and separate from your work and yourself. You stay connected and alive when finding meaning is an enduring evolution of what truly matters to you throughout the days, months, and years of your work as a clinician. While we can draw inspiration from many sources, the deepest well of personal meaning lies within us, and it is imperative to develop a path to this inner sanctum. Self-care and the personal search for a life that is meaningful are the balms that soothe, heal, and ultimately, prevent burnout. Quality of life is not just for patients; it's both an essential value and a necessity for clinicians to embrace as well as for the healthcare system to support.

The Work of the Heart: Self-Care

Authentic self-care connects us to a place of Being that transcends the external roadblocks we encounter in our lives. As clinicians, we need to care about our patients, the people we work with, and, bottom line, we need to care about ourselves. We must somehow hold on to our vulnerability so that we remain available and accessible within ourselves and with others regardless of the high demands of our work. A healing relationship needs to be open-hearted, so it's essential to be true to your authentic self and to believe in the possibility that you can stay in contact with your own humanity even in the face of inhuman circumstances. In the end, we all just want to feel that we are having a wholehearted experience of being fully alive.

Yet self-care in the healthcare setting is typically not a topic that's taught in medical school or included in ongoing training programs. The topic of self-care may be offered in a weekend workshop or a daylong course, which is adequate for the short term. However, the long-term aspect of self-care as preventive for burnout isn't introduced to students or advocated for or provided to clinicians. This lack of attention to your concerns continues into professional practice, where vulnerabilities as well as the need for personal fulfillment are infrequently considered. Self-neglect leads to both physical and emotional distress and can have serious life consequences.

Historically, it has been unacceptable for those of us in the healing profession to acknowledge our own emotional concerns, much less share that distress with others. In an interview with John Bowman from the Institute for Poetic Medicine, Jack Coulehan, physician and poet, spoke of this difficulty:

A large percentage of our medical students reflect our general culture, which is oriented toward externalities and does not promote acceptance of feelings. So there's a tendency to avoid feelings. There's a term that came out of the '50s when sociologists were studying what happened to the altruism physicians started out with in medical school, about what happened and why that disappeared later in their practice. Why did they lose this altruism when they began to connect with people's suffering. . . . What happened is that they learned to be detached. Some people said this was okay, that this was desirable. I think it is an impoverished way to look at human abilities. You don't have to be detached. It's quite possible to perform objectively and still connect with patients.[2]

It isn't 1950 anymore, yet the emotional peaks and valleys that you encounter in your work remain stigmatized, downplayed, and ignored. In the twenty-first century, it is vital to humanize the medical system to include you, the clinicians. Your voices, your stories need to be heard and accepted. How *you* feel connected with your patients and in your work matters. It's time to break the code of silent suffering and find who and what helps you.

The intense pressure that you experience when your patients are looking to you for answers can create feelings of perfectionism within you. Out of their own fear, they can demand clarity when it is not possible to give. These demands, rooted in fear and expectation, fuel the fires of perfection in an imperfect world. As a clinician, you may feel a burden to be invincible. Maintaining an image of confidence and a high level of capacity at all times, needing to be in charge so that others feel safe and secure, and attending to the needs of the patients while under duress are all part of the dynamic that breeds burnout. When the heavy load of life-and-death decisions and the image of perfection join with the sheer number of patients in treatment, a tsunami of conflicted needs is created. By accepting the realness of uncertainty in a profession that demands certainty you allow and accept your own humanness. As the psychologist Carl Rogers said, "I'm not perfect, but I'm enough."[3]

As a psychotherapist, I know that the high demands of taking care of others can leave the giver depleted unless restorative and rejuvenating choices are made. We have to acknowledge that we are human, that we are not perfect, and that we don't have all the answers. We become tired and discouraged. We feel distress and grief. We need help, too. In the psychotherapeutic world, support and consultation are not only encouraged but also deemed an essential aspect of our ongoing professional practice. My experience in working within the more traditional medical world has shown me—and sometimes shocked me—its lack of understanding and feeble consideration of the grueling hours and high expectations experienced by clinicians in these settings. I have witnessed criticism and cynicism leveled at clinicians, who often feel blamed and ignored rather than respected and held with compassion and empathy.

Who listens to you? Where do you take your sadness, anger, and fear? Do you feel that you can talk with other clinicians about difficult thoughts and feelings, or are you concerned about being judged? These are all questions that deserve deep inner contemplation as well as thoughtful discussion and active consideration within the healthcare system itself. Coping with a crazy-making system all alone is alienating and depressing. You can help your patients with the emotional distress of cancer and still find ways to include yourself in the process. It's time to break the silence of suffering, difficulty, and despair. Identifying the ways that you find help and support for your personal and professional needs is essential. A structure to reflect on these deeply individual questions is offered in the workbook section of this chapter.

I often want to give more of me than is available. What might help is shared clinic visits; another provider with whom the patient feels just as comfortable would take some of the burden off an individual provider.

—Amy Cripps, MD, oncologist, email, December, 2, 2015

The existential humanistic perspective highlights the responsibility of the clinician in making a life commitment to personal growth and renewal. The intensity of the work we have chosen requires us to take care of ourselves in order to nurture our aliveness regardless of the external pressures we deal with on a daily basis. We cannot turn our backs on ourselves. We are called on, therefore, to draw a sense of personal identity with our work and to refresh this identity as we grow as clinicians. We need to dedicate ourselves to our own growth by actively participating in a lifelong learning process while considering what our work means in the larger community that surrounds us. When who we are as beings is integrated with what we know as professionals, we create the space to be wholehearted clinicians.

Returning home to our true nature, the very center of our being, we find ourselves connected from that place inside of us to the work that we do in the outer world. This path often means a soul-searching examination of how we negotiate the familiar goals of success to which we are taught to aspire. In the process, you find yourself questioning your attachments to money, prestige, possessions, and the need for fame and fortune in favor of valuing relationships and looking at ways to simplify your life. But consider what it would take to make these changes, both individually and collectively in healthcare. What would have to shift? It seems essential to focus on humanizing the healthcare system by recognizing and validating our vulnerability as clinicians and focusing on actions that put in place some pragmatic structures and support mechanisms for support, help, and self-care for those of us who work in healthcare.

The dilemmas of addressing issues of distress, the need for support, and life and work balance for clinicians involve removing the roadblocks that are preventing their resolution. The difficulties are clear, and it is no longer enough to merely acknowledge the need to shift into a more humane system for clinicians; it is time to implement innovations in healthcare. The resistances to these needed changes are spoken to in a 2000 study, "The Painful Truth: Physicians Are Not Invincible," in which the authors stated the following:

These changes (self care, distress, support, compassion, life/work balance) will not be possible unless the current implicit definition of professional commitment and competence is challenged. Physicians need to accept the notion that professional competence allows for compassion toward other professionals and toward themselves. Recognizing distress in others, offering support and assistance to those in distress, validating the setting of appropriate limits by self and colleagues, and reducing the conflict between work life and family life could all further the cause of addressing these concerns.[4]

It is clear that continuing with the familiar old worn-out resistance to changing these perspectives is a major contributor to the halfhearted state of being known as burnout. Self-care is a preventive measure for burnout, yet often the tools that are offered only treat symptoms and do not get to the heart of the deeper need for taking care of yourself. There are levels of self-care, from activities like exercise, which relieves the momentary buildup of uncomfortable energy, and taking time off, which is great when you can take it, but this is not always possible, even when you may need it the most. Including simple, doable practices in your day-to-day life helps you to feel connected to yourself, but these coping skills sometimes don't address the real heart of the matter. They may not always be enough to take care of the real source of unhappiness. At times, it can feel like putting an ace bandage around a compound fracture. It's time to treat the wound. You will be provided with methods to help you dive into inquiry to assist you in gaining your own personal and depthful perspective on these questions in the workbook section of this chapter.

Halfhearted: Burnout

Medicine is not a job. It is not even a career. At its heart, medicine is a calling. When it comes to physician burnout, an ounce of prevention is worth a pound of cure. We must begin early in medical education to help medical students and residents explore and connect with a sense of calling to the profession. Even late in their careers, physicians need to recall that they are summoned to something older, larger, and nobler than themselves. They must never forget that a career in medicine presents one of life's greatest opportunities to become fully human through service to others.

—Richard Gunderman, "The Root of Physician Burnout"[5]

For those of you who answer the call to serve others, there can be a grave lack of recognition of your humanity. Recently, a doctor told me that the 1 hour a month she and her staff had been allotted for their wellness program, attention to self-care, reflection, and rejuvenation had been cut to 1 hour a quarter. In essence, these physicians were sent a brisk memo telling them that 4 hours a year was all that they needed when it came to their own self-care. The reason given for this cut was that physicians needed to offer more patient care.

At a conference I attended, an oncologist told the story of a sign in their physician break room that read: "Patients come first, doctors come second." The message is loud and clear for healthcare providers: You come second. It's no wonder you feel devalued. You are required to work a grueling schedule, often with a caseload numbering several thousand patients, while living under the pressure of a record-keeping system that keeps you shackled to your computer. You are a human being, and your needs are as important as those of your patients. You have a right to advocate for the support necessary to care for your humanity as well as to receive the assistance and nourishment you need to continue the work you are called to do.

We're so in demand that the pressure on us is enormous. How can we meet the needs of families without getting burned out, how to cope with that is a key challenge.

—Allison Applebaum, PhD, Director, Caregivers Clinic,
Memorial Sloan Kettering Counseling Center,
email, July 14, 2016

The statement "these changes . . . will not be possible until the current implicit definition of professional commitment and competence is challenged," from the previously mentioned study "The Painful Truth," was published in the year 2000. Twelve years later an article written by the Mayo Group and published in the *Archives of Internal Medicine* showed that 46% of 7,000 physicians surveyed felt at least one aspect of burnout.[6] Burnout symptoms were identified as emotional exhaustion, depersonalization, and low sense of personal accomplishment. Life and work balance appears to be a significant area of distress for those providing services to patients. You're usually "in the trenches," on the front line of care with no end in sight. The experience of exhaustion and stress is not isolated to a few practitioners; it is all too obviously common. As of this writing in 2017, not only are we still grappling with the issues of self-care and burnout, but also things have gotten worse, as reported in the "Medscape Lifestyle Report 2016: Bias and Burnout." In this study, 46% of oncology professionals reported suffering from burnout, and the severity rating of burnout in oncology moved to third position, beneath those professionals in critical care and neurology, at 4.40 on a scale of 1–7.[7]

[2016's] Medscape survey, echoing other recent national surveys, strongly suggests that burnout among US physicians has reached a critical level. Burnout in these surveys is defined as loss of enthusiasm for work, feelings of cynicism, and a low sense of personal accomplishment. Of note, however, burnout rates for all specialties are higher this year. The 2015 survey published in the Mayo Clinic Proceedings compared burnout between 2011 and 2014 and observed an increase in the percentage of physicians reporting at least one burnout symptom, from 45.5% to 54.4%.

—Carol Peckham, "Medscape Lifestyle Report"[8]

The percentages of burnout for women is usually, and not surprisingly, higher for females in healthcare than for their male counterparts. The bar is set very high for women when it comes to being acknowledged as competent in healthcare. They toil for lower salaries and fewer academic promotions. All of these factors point to a higher burnout rate for women in healthcare.

A 2016 study led by researchers at the Harvard T. H. Chan School of Public Health reported that elderly hospital patients fare better when treated by female physicians. Senior author and Harvard professor Dr. Ashish Jha, Director of the Harvard Global Health Institute, summed up the results: "We found that when patients are hospitalized, when they receive care from a female physician, they're more likely to survive, and they're less likely to come back, than when their doctor is a man."[9] Research also found that female doctors tend to be more effective at communicating with patients, and this most certainly is a factor in quality of care for people regardless of survival or longevity.

However, statistics show a higher rate of burnout for women in health-care. Female doctors' patients live longer, but the doctors are still paid 8% less than male colleagues.[10] While there is an acknowledgment in health-care for the truth that a woman must work much harder to prove the quality of her work and to receive the recognition she has earned, these issues remain unaddressed in any solution-based manner that would in-volve professional acknowledgment and equal financial compensation. To this day, the work of the female professional is still viewed as less valuable than that of their male counterparts, as evidenced in the females receiving less respect, less recognition, and lower compensation (Figure 6.1).

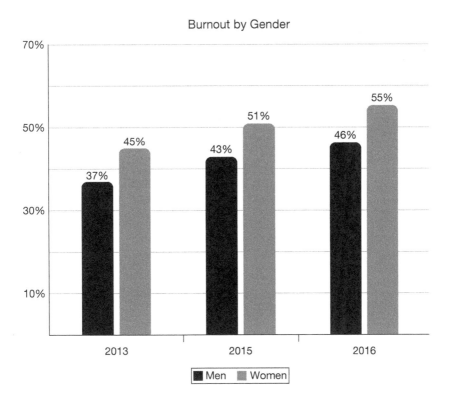

FIGURE 6.1

Burnout by gender.

In this year's Medscape lifestyle survey, as in previous years, more female physicians (55%) expressed burnout than their male peers (46%). Of note, however, these percentages have trended up for both men and women since this question was first asked in Medscape's 2013 survey. In that year, 45% of women and 37% of men reported burnout.[11]

Female or male, when you are disengaged within yourself and in your work you begin to live a half-hearted life. The essence of burnout is this lack of engagement, a strong sense of alienation that is in contrast with working and living wholeheartedly. If you are experiencing burnout, it's likely that the root of your pain is deeper than a surface wound. It may involve how fairly—or unfairly—you feel you are being compensated and how connected you feel with the work you are doing and the people you serve. In the end, how connected you feel within yourself is the foundation of your personal satisfaction. Making an ongoing commitment to your well-being first as who you are and second as a clinician is a way to affirm your own worth as well as a method to ensure your work satisfaction. Most importantly, it creates a practice of self-love that can carry you through rough seas. You can develop ongoing systems and processes that support you in both your work and your life. As these practices are profoundly personal, the modes of care will change throughout your life, just as your needs and wants shift and are not static in nature. The workbook section offers you a structure that you can use again and again as a method of self-discovery that encourages you to attend to yourself in meaningful ways.

Adjustment to a system that is killing your spirit is not an acceptable solution to the serious problem of burnout. Learning how to take care of yourself within that system while demanding that changes be made to better accommodate your needs are worthy and necessary endeavors. Our concerns for our own well-being and the successful longevity of our work as clinicians depends on giving serious relevance to addressing the issues of our quality of life head-on. We need to question the parts of ourselves that have turned away from these concerns and, thus, allowed the healthcare system to neglect the problems that lead to the experience of burnout. When we abandon ourselves, we feel lost. That is the time when you need to ask yourself, What is the part of me that turns away from myself? Spending time in reflection and self-inquiry helps you to remember what first called you to your work and what now keeps you present and still growing as you listen to the voice of that call as it is alive in you today.

Wholehearted: Finding Meaning

I am not what happened to me, I am what I choose to become.

—Carl Jung[12]

Your personal and professional well-being depends on your commitment to an ongoing practice of reflection that helps you to continue discovering what truly matters to you. With this promise to yourself, you honor your own deeply personal, always unfolding search for meaning. Your commitment to the exploration of who you are beneath and beyond the familiar external goals of what is considered successful allows you to enter through the gates of self-discovery to a deeper inner place of awareness. Finding meaning in our work is an always-evolving process, and it is in this continuous searching that we often surprise and revive ourselves from a stale, rote way of work that results in us going through the motions and merely performing tasks. This lifelong path of education, personal development, and growth is not about reaching a specific destination. Indeed, we often get to where we think we wanted to be only to discover that we are merely at another fork in the road of our lives. This is the ever-awakening nature of becoming ourselves and then bringing that self forward into our lives.

So how do we attain access to the gateways to our inner world? Most of us aren't taught how to develop a practice of reflection known as inward searching.[13] In fact, we are often discouraged from the quieter internal path in favor of the pursuit of external goals and endeavors. Yet when we bring awareness to our concerns and ask the important question regarding what matters to us, we gain the clarity we need to move forward from our own authentic perspective. Developing the capacity for inward searching helps to identify the roadblocks that get in our way of satisfaction, validates the power of genuine presence, and creates a structure for us to take our needs and wants seriously. We need to be willing to explore our own feelings, beliefs, and values to remain in touch with ourselves in meaningful ways. There are numerous paths that you can take on your journey of reflection and self-awareness, and it will be absolutely essential to find those that resonate with you. Meditation and different types of contemplative practice, psychotherapy, the expressive arts, and time in nature are all methods of deep self-discovery. The questions in the workbook section are designed to assist you in finding ways that work for you, and a resource guide is also provided.

Meaning is, of course, personal to each of us. It doesn't always have to be *meaning*; there is a great deal to be said for the moments of our lives that are unexpectedly beautiful in their simplicity and spontaneity. It can be easy to miss the power of small moments when our minds become so busy that we are not present and paying attention to what is right in front of us. The type of intention I'm talking about doesn't involve the usual to-do list but is an engaged way of being in touch with the unexpected instances of genuineness that surround us. An ongoing exploration of our being brings about a more expansive intuitiveness that greatly adds to the quality of our lives by helping us be more connected with ourselves and with others.

Being in contact within ourselves while also extending an invitation for others to be in contact with us is a primary way to extinguish a sense of isolation. Staying connected with our work is one of the greatest challenges of a career in healthcare. While we did not have the experience, the skills, or the clinical expertise when we started out, we came to our work with fresh eyes and an open heart that wanted to serve and help others. Over the years, it's all too easy to fall into a jaded and dissatisfied state of mind due to tiredness, overwork, and disillusionment. We can lose touch with why we came to our work in the first place.

Continued attention to the care of your emotional resilience is another part of making meaning a focus. Dealing with trauma is inherent in our work, and we can become dragged down in these heartbreaks and distresses without even noticing that we have lost touch with our vulnerability and have grown numb. This numbness threatens the link to why we are even doing the work that we do. Therefore, it is important to find restorative practices that offer a deeper and more expansive level of self-care, practices that feed your heart and soul and bolster your emotional resilience.

Deeply resting, fully playing, and enjoying intellectual stimulation are more than coping mechanisms, as they lead us in exploring a deeper layer of self-care that involves our innermost perspective in all parts of creating a meaningful life that support the often stressful situations of our clinical work. These are aspects of ourselves that are more long term in nature, sometimes even including our deepest values and life intentions. Your needs in each of these categories will change over the course of your life, so it's helpful to keep an open mind and be willing to explore multiple options and stretch yourself in new directions. Follow through is even more imperative when you feel too tired to bother to check out things that interest and move you beyond your comfortable, but perhaps disconnected, state of being. The workbook section addresses both short-term and long-term intentions by giving you suggestions and a narrative template for use with your own contemplation.

The bottom line is that we are responsible for creating our own meaning. An existential viewpoint of personal responsibility as a clinician highlights continued recognition and focus on accepting and dealing with life's realities as they exist. Springing from this bottom line is the need for us to attend to our experience as we deal with the existential issues in our work. This requires identifying with our work and recognizing when this identity feels disconnected. We also need to make a lifelong vow to our own professional development and personal awareness as a means of support for a strong, ethical personal standard of quality. All of this speaks to setting long-term intentions, which, as the years and changes of your life occur, shift and grow and remain a place of aliveness and exploration.

Setting a long-term intention is like setting the compass of our heart. No matter how rough the storms, how difficult the terrain, even if we have to backtrack around obstacles, our direction is clear. The fruits of dedication are visible in the best of human endeavors.

—Jack Kornfield, *The Wise Heart*[14]

Setting the intentions that allow you to find what is meaningful to you is a deeply personal act of consciousness. The workbook section of this chapter is designed to give you a structure for your thoughts, feelings, and reflections. Give yourself the time and space to explore what fulfillment means to you. The questions are posed to encourage you to return to them on a regular basis in order to continue your ongoing commitment to self-care, the prevention of burnout, and finding meaning.

For me, balancing my life with a variety of activities is very important. In order to restore myself and my energy and really show up for others, I need time to get out of my head and out of my feelings, and I do this by making art, swimming, dancing, being with friends, therapy.

—Merideth Shamszad, MFT, email, July 3, 2016

Part I: Questions

- What support do *you* need?

  _____

  _____

  _____

  _____

- How well do you feel supported by others in your work?

  _____

  _____

  _____

  _____

- List the ways in which you take care of yourself.

  _____

  _____

  _____

  _____

- Do you feel that your attention to your own self-care is working? How? And if not, what do you believe you need to do differently?

  _____

  _____

  _____

  _____

- What does rest mean to you? List some ways that help you to feel rested.

  _____

  _____

  _____

  _____

- How do you play? What is fun to you? Think about how you bring enjoyment into your life and what you might want to add to those good times.

_____

_____

_____

_____

- What stimulates your mind? How, where, and with whom do you get the intellectual and creative stimulation that feeds you?

_____

_____

_____

_____

- How do you nurture yourself? Think about the people and the activities that you associate with feeling fulfilled. Who are they? What are they?

_____

_____

_____

_____

- How would you rate the level of stress that you experience in your work? Use a scale of 1 to 10, with 10 being the highest level of stress. Write down your thoughts and feelings.

_____

_____

_____

_____

- What is the most difficult part of your work?

_____

_____

■ Do you sometimes feel disconnected from your work? In what ways?

_____

_____

_____

_____

■ List some of the ways that help you feel connected.

_____

_____

_____

_____

■ Do you experience feelings of isolation in your workplace? What do you need to feel a sense of belonging?

_____

_____

_____

_____

■ Reflect on your need for contact and write your thoughts and feelings.

_____

_____

_____

_____

■ What are the most rewarding aspects of your work?

_____

_____

_____

_____

- What are your signs of burnout? How do you think you can become more aware of the early signs as a preventive measure? List the signs, how you can notice when they occur, and the ways you can treat them early.

_____

_____

_____

_____

- Do you think that support groups, psychotherapy, retreats, and workshops are helpful resources for you as a provider in dealing with isolation and burnout? Do you find that you have viable options and choices in these areas? What would you like to see offered as a resource for you?

_____

_____

_____

_____

- What are the most difficult pressures you experience in terms of providing survivorship care? What would assist you in the delivery of the care plans? What would support you in the work that you do?

_____

_____

_____

_____

- What types of resources do you need to be able to include the emotional care of your patients into a treatment plan? Would you be open to integrating a psychotherapist or social worker in your practice to discuss the survivorship care plan with your patients?

_____

_____

_____

_____

- Do you have an adequate referral system to provide to those patients who request or need help in dealing with the emotional difficulties of a cancer diagnosis? Do you have someone in your practice who can handle this for you?

_____

_____

_____

_____

- What do you find most meaningful about your work?

_____

_____

_____

_____

- Do you have an ongoing relationship with finding meaning in the work that you do?

_____

_____

_____

_____

- How comfortable are you with your vulnerability in your professional life?

_____

_____

_____

_____

- Do you have a practice of self-reflection? How do you search within yourself?

_____

_____

■ What touches you in the small moments of your life?

_____

_____

_____

_____

■ Do you feel like you make a difference? How and in what ways?

_____

_____

_____

_____

Part II: Short-Term and Long-Term Intentions

By reflecting on what you have discovered using these questions, you can create your own survivorship plan to help you continue to be personally healthy as well as to work effectively. The nature of your work involves the reality of ongoing stress and requires you to be an advocate for yourself. Looking at the difficulties in your work as well as at the rewards shows you important factors that can help you in this endeavor. As you take yourself into the heart of your choice to heal others, you remember who you are.

The next section is divided into two parts: short-term and long-term intentions. Short-term intentions help you focus on who you are now in your life, while long-term intentions aid you in making plans for the future based on what you deeply value in the bigger picture of your life. This exploration helps you to consider your quality of life as it is essential for your ongoing well-being in the work that you do.

Quality of life in previous chapters, as defined by the University of Toronto Quality of Life Research Institute (http://sites.utoronto.ca/qol/

qol_model.htm), is "the degree to which a person enjoys the important possibilities of his or her life. Possibilities result from the opportunities and limitations each person has in his/her life and reflect the interaction of personal and environmental factors. Three major life domains are identified: Being, Belonging, and Becoming." Your definition of quality of life is uniquely your own and extremely personal, so I encourage you to spend time exploring what is truly meaningful to you in your life.

Think of this as a narrative. Imagine that you are being asked the questions and then respond as if you were having a dialogue with another person. You may want to imagine speaking to a colleague or an associate in your field. You may think of a friend, therapist, or spiritual advisor. Perhaps you feel most comfortable having this dialogue with yourself. Don't worry about right or wrong answers because they don't exist.

Keep a copy of these plans and update them periodically as what works for you changes with your needs and wants at different times in your life. Self-advocacy in terms of self-care is essential and needs to contain physical, emotional, mental, and spiritual/meaningful components in order to be integrative. Create a care plan that is visible to you each day. You may write it down so that you can see it, keep it on your computer or in your phone.

Short-Term Intentions

Short-term intentions can take the pressure off of thinking that you need to know what you want before you find where you are in the present moment. Slow down and release the tension you put on yourself to perform and work beyond what is healthy for you. Initially, short-term intentions may look like taking small breaks during your workday by reading a book, walking around the block to get some fresh air, or spending more time with friends and family. They are simple and don't require a lot of planning and work. In short, they are easy. While these intentions involve work, family, relationships, creative projects, travel, and other things that may take some planning, remember that they are flexible and, in that way, doable.

Write down some of your short-term intentions.

_____

_____

_____

_____

Long-Term Intentions

Long-term intentions require self-inquiry into what you value and what is most important to you in the bigger picture of your life. A good question to ask yourself is, What really matters to me? Sit with this question, search within yourself in an open space of awareness, and watch what emerges without judgment. Allow yourself to be in a place of self-discovery so that you can thoughtfully choose your life plan based on who you are.

Long-term intentions may involve education, work and career pursuits, creative projects, relationships and intimacy with others, and attending to the connection you have with yourself. This search is not necessarily motivated by external circumstances or materialistic pursuits, yet both of these areas may be included in your plan. It is important to value this aspect of long-term intention without getting caught up in how productive or practical it *should* be. Both the inner and outer world are a part of this exploration. Allow yourself the space and time to be with this inquiry without pressing for quick answers. Be sure that you are paying attention to what really matters to you.

Write down some of your long-term intentions.

_____

_____

_____

_____

Your care is as important as the person you are caring for.

—Cheryl Krauter

Resources

We can always find a moment to slow down and tune into ourselves. It may only be for a minute, but in that minute we affirm our ongoing commitment to our own well-being. The following resources are meant as suggestions for you to explore. I recommend that you pay attention to the resources that draw you in and then follow that interest to see where it may take you.

I. Mobile apps can help you when you're on the go and need a moment to check in with yourself.
- Stress Doctor by Azumio, Incorporated—Stress reducer and slow-breathing yoga exercise
  http://www.azumio.com/
- Breathe2Relax
  http://t2health.dcoe.mil/apps/breathe2relax
- Calm
  https://www.calm.com/
- Headspace: Guided Meditation and Mindfulness by Headspace Meditation Limited
  https://www.headspace.com/
- Smiling Mind by Smiling Mind
  https://www.smilingmind.com.au/
- Mindfulness Daily by Inward, Incorporated
  http://www.mindfulnessdailyapp.com/

II. Fitness breaks you can take while you are working
- Mayo Clinic Adult Health Online
  https://www.mayoclinic.org/healthy-lifestyle/adult-health/in-depth/office-stretches/art-20046041?pg=2
- Yoga for Healthy Aging
  http://yogaforhealthyaging.blogspot.com
- Get outside, even if it's just for a few minutes
- Remember to eat
- Make contact with others

III. CDs to help you unwind and reconnect with yourself when you get home
- *The Wise Heart* by Jack Kornfield
  https://www.soundstrue.com/store/audio/the-wise-heart-4089.html

- *Guided Meditations for Self-Healing: Essential Practices to Relieve Physical and Emotional Suffering and Enhance Recovery* by Jack Kornfield
  https://www.soundstrue.com/store/audio/guided-meditations-for-self-healing-1744.html
- CDs by Jon Kabat-Zinn
  https://www.mindfulnesscds.com/collections/cds
- *Finding True Refuge: Meditations for Difficult Times* by Tara Brach
  https://www.soundstrue.com/store/audio/finding-true-refuge-3000.html
- *The Healthy Mind Platter* by Dan Seigel, MD
  http://www.drdansiegel.com/resources/healthy_mind_platter/
- *What to Remember When Waking* by David Whyte
  http://davidwhyte.stores.yahoo.net/whtorewhwa6c.html

Notes

1. John Stone, Gaudeamus Igitur, written for the commencement ceremony of Emory University's School of Medicine, 1982. Music from *Apartment 8: New and Selected Poems*, LSU Press, Baton Rouge, LA, 2004, p. 102. Reprinted with permission of Louisana State Press.
2. Jack Coulehan, MD, interview by John Bowman, *Changing the World: Arts and Medicine*, The Institute for Poetic Medicine, Palo Alto, CA, n.d., p. 3. http://www.poeticmedicine.org/jack-coulehan.html.
3. Carl Rogers, Quotable Quote. Good Reads. n.d. http://www.goodreads.com/quotes/411730-i-m-not-perfect-but-i-m-enough.
4. Merry N. Miller, MD, and K. Ramsey Mcgowen, PhD, The Painful Truth: Physicians Are Not Invincible. *South Med J*. 2000;93(10):8. https://www.ncbi.nlm.nih.gov/pubmed/11147478.
5. Richard Gunderman, The Root of Physician Burnout. *The Atlantic*, August 27, 2012, p. 6.
6. T. D. Shanafelt, S. Boone, L. Tan, et al., Burnout and Satisfaction with Work-Life Balance Among US Physicians Relative to the General US Population. *Arch Intern Med*. 2012;172(18):11377.
7. Carol Peckham, Medscape Lifestyle Report 2016: Bias and Burnout. https://www.medscape.com/slideshow/lifestyle-2016-overview-6007335. Published January 13, 2016.
8. Peckham, Medscape Lifestyle Report 2016.

9. Carey Goldberg, Harvard Study: Elderly Hospital Patients Live Longer, Do Better With Female Doctors. *CommonHealth*. December 19, 2016, p. 2.

10. Peckham, Medscape Lifestyle Report 2016.

11. Peckham, Medscape Lifestyle Report 2016.

12. Carl Jung, Quotable Quote. Good Reads. n.d. https://www.goodreads.com/quotes/50795-i-am-not-what-happened-to-me-i-am-what.

13. Bugental, James F. T., *Psychotherapy and Process: The Fundamentals of an Existential-Humanistic Approach*, Addison-Wesley, Boston, 1978, p. 51.

14. Jack Kornfield, *The Wise Heart: A Guide to the Universal Teachings of Buddhist Psychology*, Bantam Dell, Division of Random House, New York, 2008, p. 261.

Some old men came to see Abba Poemen, and said to him: Tell us, when we see our brothers dozing during the sacred office, should we pinch them so they will stay awake? The old man said to them: Actually, if I saw a brother sleeping, I would put his head on my knees and let him rest.

—Desert Fathers, *Stories of the Spirit, Stories of the Heart*[1]

One of the biggest blessings we have is our connections to colleagues who become our friends at work. Most people can all name at least one person who has been an invaluable partner and support person at work. I've been fortunate to work with collaborative groups and to experience the satisfaction of unique and creative forces working together as a team; in talking to other clinicians, this is always something people mention when they talk about the positive side of work and where they feel supported. We carry a burden of concern in our work, which is why down-to-earth and caring collegial relationships can bring us back from the edges of these daily concerns and relentless self-doubts that go hand in hand with the caring professions. They can help us find ourselves when we feel lost.

As a psychotherapist, I have worked in adolescent group homes, in treatment facilities for the severally mentally ill, at a crisis unit in a hospital, as an adjunct professor, as a clinical supervisor in a graduate psychology program, and for nearly 40 years as a solo practitioner in a private psychotherapy practice. My work with cancer survivors has led me to become involved with a community cancer center, cancer healthcare, and survivorship committees in both community and hospital settings. In these institutions, often known as "the trenches," the dedicated professionals comprise the staff; decades after working with them, many are still my closest friends. There's a special bond forged when you're working in dramatic, heartbreaking, and often dangerous situations. When we work in life-and-death situations, we're called on to think fast and move quickly, all the while keeping an open mind and heart to our patients. What has always saved me in the intensity of all of these positions were the people who worked alongside me. During my time at the crisis unit, my colleagues were an intelligent and funny group of people who could have had a successful stint on *Saturday Night Live*. Laughter created a way to let go of horror, grief, and an exhaustion that could cut deep into the bones at times.

Over my many years of work, I have been fortunate to have been part of numerous consultation groups and organizations that existed for the purpose of keeping us alive as clinicians. I have been a part of an on-going consultation group since 1988, and it's those people who know me, as I know them, in some of the deepest, most substantive ways imaginable. As a group, we continue to support one another through both professional and personal trials and tribulations. The comfort of being known for your strengths as well as being accepted for that which challenges you is an antidote for feelings of isolation in clinical work. Shining a light of awareness on what is working and what is not working leads us out of those dark inner places that are so easy to collapse into in that long haul of our work as clinicians.

As my involvement in cancer healthcare has deepened, I have become more aware of a serious disconnection between clinicians working within the system. Given my own good experiences on this front, I'm concerned by our healthcare system, which does not recognize the need for clinicians to support one another in order to address the serious problem of burnout. The usual excuses for this lack of collegial inter-action revolve around no time and not enough money. These antiquated beliefs are simply not true; we can always find the time to connect with one another, and it doesn't have to cost anything. Cancer healthcare needs to value the people who work within its system. Like the patients, the clinicians aren't merely numbers. In 2017, I attended a large on-cology conference and was struck by the tense and harried atmosphere of the group and its attendees. Most of the discussions around the difficulties of providing patient care focused on time and money, with very little dialogue involving the human side of patient care. Perhaps I "missed the memo," but I did not come across talks or workshops on collaboration between clinicians for the purpose of supporting both their professional and their personal well-being.

If the environment discourages open communication, you won't do it.
It's not a priority. We need to voice the need for consultation and peer
supervision.

—Allison Applebaum, PhD, email, July 14, 2016

This drives home for me how much we need to value the importance of our relationships with one another and speak out within the healthcare system, giving voice to the need for attention to the importance of collaboration among clinicians. In their book *Patient Safety and Quality*, Michelle O'Daniel and Alan H. Rosenstein wrote the following:

It is important to point out that fostering a team collaboration
environment may have hurdles to overcome: additional time; perceived
loss of autonomy; lack of confidence or trust in decisions of others; clashing
perceptions; territorialism; and lack of awareness of one provider of the
education, knowledge, and skills held by colleagues from other disciplines
and professions.[2]

They report that "improved teamwork and communication are described by healthcare workers as among the most important factors in improving clinical effectiveness and job satisfaction."[3]

Table 7.1 lists some of the common barriers found in establishing meaningful collaboration. However, it's important to view these barriers to strong collegial connections not as a predicament that cannot be solved but as a challenge that can be overcome with commitment and open communication.

TABLE 7.1

Common Barriers to Interprofessional Communication and Collaboration

- Personal values and expectations
- Personality differences
- Hierarchy
- Disruptive behavior
- Culture and ethnicity
- Generational differences
- Gender
- Historical interprofessional and intraprofessional rivalries
- Differences in language and jargon

- Differences in schedules and professional routines
- Varying levels of preparation, qualifications, and status
- Differences in requirements, regulations, and norms of professional education
- Fears of diluted professional identity
- Differences in accountability, payment, and rewards
- Concerns regarding clinical responsibility
- Complexity of care
- Emphasis on rapid decision-making

Source: From Professional Communication and Team Collaboration.[4] Reprinted with permission of the Agency for Healthcare Research and Quality.

Table 7.1 may make our challenges seem harder to overcome, but when we adopt a humanistic, person-centered approach to cancer healthcare, we become aware of the stereotypical ways that we identify ourselves and one another, and in that awareness we can choose more clear and open ways of communication. In essence, we become human beings with one another, people who are bonding together for a common cause. Issues of gender, culture and ethnicity, and generational differences are complex and deep seated and, because of this complexity, often more difficult to work through. However, none of these differences should imply resignation, but instead should encourage us to move forward and do the hard work of looking at how we can change dated stereotypes and biases. It is not enough to settle for the status quo in today's world; we must dig deep and work with one another toward a metamorphosis in how we hold diversity. Any topic on this list can be shifted in the service of wholehearted collaboration between clinicians.

How Self-Care of Clinicians Is Sacrificed in the Service of the Patient

The majority of the material on collaboration among clinicians is aimed at clinical collaboration in the service of taking care of patients. The traditional viewpoint that holds that clinicians need to come from a place of detachment in their work has leaked into the realm of their collegial relationships and created distance among those who could offer a great deal to one another. The message of "patient first, doctor second" is rooted in these outworn traditions of self-sacrifice, attitudes that are no longer serving us. We need to head down a different path together.

Just as life-threatening illness is a great equalizer among patients, so is the emotional distress of clinicians in institutions, out in the community, or in private practice. Our human wants and needs transcend the differences in our disciplines and circumstances and call on us to join together to take care of one another. Self-care is an essential responsibility of each of us as individuals and no less a worthy endeavor in the service of the well-being of all than is the care of others. We do not exist alone in our work; we are not soloists. Indeed, each of us is a violin, a horn, or a bass playing our own individual note in a bigger symphony. When we acknowledge how important we are to one another, we enter a place that is larger than ourselves and form a bond of collaboration and care. In times of exhaustion and despair, we are lit by the light of one another's companionship.

Collaboration is about supporting one another, enhancing each other's work, encouraging personal and professional growth, positively confronting one another during difficult times, and celebrating each other's triumphs. The intention of compassionate and connected collegial relationships is to create harmony, as well as to open up avenues of fluidity, change, and openness with one another and in the work that we do. These supportive work relationships create a way to build cooperation and give us the honor of having each other's backs. There is great power when a community of people care about one another and express that in their actions and interactions. We experience high levels of satisfaction and happiness when we care about the well-being of others.

Team-based care and professional collaborations are often inextricably connected with the goal of patient care. Obviously, this is key to establishing a patient-centered healthcare system. However, the focus on patient care, while essential, cannot negate the heartfelt attention clinicians need and must have to thrive. Collaboration in service of patient care was covered in Chapter 2; in this chapter, we explore a more intimate viewpoint, one that supports forming an alliance between clinicians, for the purpose of opening a conversation that revolves around person-centered care that is inclusive of the clinicians.

A team approach to patient care is especially important in cancer care because each member of the team contributes their own expertise and experience.

—Dr. Jon Greif, email, July 20, 2016

The need for personal support in the clinical world has long been kept in a dark, silent room of shame where we are instructed to hide our needs and practice detachment from our thoughts and feelings. We are encouraged to pretend that our vulnerability does not exist. These archaic views of selflessness and "rugged individualism" still prevail throughout the healthcare system, making it difficult for clinicians to turn to one another when they are hurting. The message is that emotional detachment is the way we survive in clinical practice. With the astounding rise of burnout indicating that clinicians feel isolated and alienated, nothing could be further from the truth. This same edict has also caused us to turn a blind eye when we observe a colleague in distress. The code of "strong at all costs" has also prevented us from reaching out to our colleagues when we are in a tough spot, which is basically self-harmful and, in the end, far from "cost-effective." In reality, we're all working without a net, and the sooner we acknowledge that we live in a vulnerable and uncertain place, the sooner we can begin to act as a net for one another. In the words of Charles Darwin, "In the long history of humankind (and animal kind, too) those who learned to collaborate and improvise most effectively have prevailed."[5]

When we invite a conversation with our colleagues, we open the possibility of the power of supporting our shared experience. Courageous conversations involve things that really matter to us—our concerns, difficulties, and triumphs. We learn about others by being curious and showing an interest in who another person is, not just in what they do. When we know the people we are shoulder to shoulder with in our work, we can also recognize when they are in trouble. We can turn to them when we are in trouble. We can create a spacious atmosphere that allows for an open dialogue. Open communication, in and of itself, builds a foundation of concern between people that frees space for authentic disclosure and brings empathy into the realities of our stressful clinical work. We can become allies in a common cause and learn to spot distress in our colleagues rather than letting them drown.

The possibilities of work partnerships are endless as we form alliances that can last a lifetime.

How We Can Trust and Depend on One Another

Lean on me, when you're not strong
And I'll be your friend
I'll help you carry on
For it won't be long
Till I'm gonna need
Somebody to lean on

—Bill Withers, "Lean on Me"[6]

Each of us, in our separate roles and disciplines, has our own contribution and a set of unique skills to bring to patient care. This diversity, along with our individual gifts (and quirks), is what makes us unique and valuable as clinicians working together. Our professional competency will grow and evolve over time as we progress from being beginners to masters of our work. We advance from insecure professionals relying on textbooks and the generalized use of tools and techniques into intuitive clinicians who have the capacity to think outside the box and offer creative perspectives. That said, I believe that no matter how long we have been in our practices, every new day and each new patient brings us back to being a beginner in whatever we are facing in any given moment. It takes willingness to acknowledge what we don't know to learn and collaborate with colleagues throughout our lives.

Collaboration in healthcare is often looked at in terms of clinicians assuming complementary roles in order to work cooperatively and share the responsibilities of problem-solving and decision-making in order to effectively care for patients. This elementary structure, while important, does not cover the complexities that arise between clinicians that can block satisfying relationships. Meaningful interactions depend on a level of personal awareness and responsibility. In person-centered care, this means that we cannot just follow a suggested script; we must be able to communicate from a conscious place within ourselves. This type of communication places a value on authenticity and a genuine recognition of the person you are interacting with; in order to be as fully present as you can be, you need to continue to commit to your own personal development.

One of the biggest roadblocks to this aware and authentic mode of communication is the hierarchical structures embedded in the healthcare system. How do we address these structures that clearly exist and create a separation among practitioners that causes both personal pain and professional divisiveness? This is a complicated question that requires us to risk letting down our guard and moving beyond the familiar roles that we hide behind in our work. People become stuck in stereotypical roles defined by their titles or license type and caught by unspoken rules about crossing over certain rigid professional borders, which causes rifts that affect how we join together in effective and meaningful connections. I have experienced professional interactions where I felt patronized because of my master's level degree, which is sometimes greeted as inadequate, denying the length and depth of my 40-year career as a psychotherapist. I know without a doubt that I have been taken less seriously and even dismissed by professionals who only look at the role and the degree behind the name. I have talked to numerous clinicians who have also been treated this way within the existing hierarchical systems.

Kathleen M. Sutcliffe, PhD, Elizabeth Lewton, PhD, MPH, and Marilynn M. Rosenthal, PhD, acknowledged these hierarchical realities in their research:

Communication failures in the medical setting arise from vertical hierarchical differences, concerns with upward influence, role conflict, and ambiguity and struggles with interpersonal power and conflict. Communication is likely to be distorted or withheld in situations where there are hierarchical differences between two communicators, particularly when one person is concerned about appearing incompetent, does not want to offend the other, or perceives that the other is not open to communication.[7]

The Sutcliffe et al. report clearly pointed out an environment of fear that is preventing clinicians from having open and clear communication with one another. In an interview, a therapist who works in a community agency told me, "We need to leave the competition at the door and give one another permission to speak freely without fear of being blamed or judged." An oncologist answered my question on the need for collaboration with these thoughts: "I think it's crucial and not done enough. It's difficult to know how to approach a difficult colleague, a colleague who is a friend, a colleague who has made a mistake. There needs to be a better forum for discussion, one that includes social workers, therapists, etc." In an interview, the program director of a hospital survivorship program responded by saying, "I think it is still the old boys network in many places. There should be supportive sessions for providers where they get tips from those who are role models for good communication." These three examples from clinicians in varied disciplines and in different settings all indicate the need and the desire to have more effective and collaborative communication between practitioners in a safe and respectful atmosphere.

In order to truly work collaboratively, we need to learn about the individual roles of others, separate the role from the person, and find ways to interface with other clinicians effectively. These arbitrary barriers can be overcome with an open attitude, feelings of mutual respect and trust, and the acknowledgment that we all have something of value to bring to the table.

On a personal level, actually taking the time to know the people you work with makes for more engaged and meaningful work relationships and leads to stronger feelings of belonging. You can choose how intimate you want to be, and not everyone will be your best friend, but knowing more about your colleagues' expertise, backgrounds, and values and understanding their particular knowledge all build successful work partnerships. When someone becomes a real person to us, not just somebody who inhabits a professional role, we are freed up to relate to them in ways that are far more connected and supportive. Professional boundaries are important up to a point, but they can too easily become prison walls, pushing people away and keeping you enclosed in a space of solitary confinement. Little to no harm has ever occurred during friendly and concerned interactions where we feel treated like human beings.

When clinicians do not feel supported by one another, it creates a wasteland that lacks a certain generosity of spirit. This lack of collaborative relationship alienates us from creating caring environments that promote and encourage healing interactions between clinicians of all disciplines.

Sometimes, we forget that we are all on the home team and that, regardless of our differences, we are playing the same game. We will experience a sense of lack and feelings of impoverishment when we stray too far from recognizing the value of relationship. We will forget that we need to matter to others and to let others matter to us. We do better when we join together in compassion on the journey that we travel with one another. Giving of ourselves does not take anything away from us or make us less. Rather, when we give of ourselves and receive from others we are filled up from being in connection.

Seeing and experiencing our colleagues as vulnerable human beings allows us to open up and trust them with our concerns and confidences. The foundation of trust is respect and recognition, and when we feel this with others we can depend on them. Regardless of the clinical language that we speak, we can transcend the harmful patterns of exclusivity and form inclusive work partnerships. Leaving behind the familiar and safe jargon of our individual clinical roles, we begin communicating with each other as human beings with common and often universal needs, wants, and values. We can learn to create a common language that joins us together and releases old barriers that get in the way of a kind of deep compassion for each other that builds healing collegial relationships and benefits effective teamwork.

Keep it simple. Thoughtful communication does not have to be that complicated when we make a commitment to an open-minded and open-hearted stance in our relationships. Take a moment to slow down. Believe that those around you want to be their best and do good work. Step aside from proving your point and listen to what others have to say. Do the best you can to be present in all situations. This basic humanistic mode of communication adopts a holistic approach to the shared realities of our essential human existence and opens myriad possibilities for an integrative and relational base of collaborative communication. A humanistic attitude will help to bypass being stuck in times of chaos and conflict and has the potential to turn difficult interactions and problems into creative and satisfying moments. Our interactions run more smoothly when we come from a place of recognizing our mutual, elementary need for love and respect.

All have their worth and each contributes to the worth of the others.

—J. R. R. Tolkien, *The Silmarillion*[8]

The depth of a truly collegial relationship does not depend on length of acquaintance. I have worked meaningfully with clinicians with whom I have spent less than an entire hour, and I have been in continual consultation with people I have known for nearly 40 years. I have consulted by telephone with people who I have never met in person and developed deep and meaningful connections. The clinical teams I have been a part of have given me a wealth of knowledge that I greatly appreciate and provided me with a feeling of camaraderie that is invaluable. I believe that you have also had the refreshing and inspiring experience of being part of a collaborative team and enjoyed the rewards that a powerful alliance can provide. As human beings, we are relational in our very being; we need one another. This is not trivial in our work together as clinicians, it is not an elective; it is an inherent human need to trust and depend on one another. Genuine connection with one another doesn't just happen automatically; our relationships need to be nurtured in order for them to grow. Forming work alliances needs to be a conscious concern that we give attention to on a regular basis. As the level of fear between clinicians declines and is replaced by an atmosphere of safety, a more compassionate, person-focused culture emerges.

Mentoring

In order to be a mentor, and an effective one, one must care. You must care. You don't have to know how many square miles are in Idaho, you don't need to know what is the chemical makeup of chemistry, or of blood or water. Know what you know and care about the person, care about what you know and care about the person you're sharing with.

—Maya Angelou[9]

Recently, a young physician told me that she was struggling with issues of communication and collaboration at work. As we talked about her distress, she told me she wanted and needed "established, experienced physicians to help her find her way by sharing their own experiences." What she was talking about was mentorship, and she was longing for it.

Mentoring younger professionals is the responsibility of those of us who have walked the road ahead of them. Mentoring another clinician differs from a supervisory position, where you are required to assess someone's skills and rate their work performance. Mentors and mentees create a relationship that becomes a safe place to discuss sensitive subjects, concerns, personal distresses, as well as successes, without a fear that the conversation will be shared with others or viewed as some kind of proof of incompetence or inadequacy.

A successful mentoring relationship not only provides support but also offers a framework for the mentee to grow and develop both personally and professionally. A humanistic approach allows the young clinician to explore and discover who they are in their work, not who they feel they should be (or how you feel they should be). In this way, they have a head start on remaining connected within themselves and establishing a foundation of personal exploration and self-care that will promote their path of lifelong learning.

When done well, mentoring is both a gratifying and a demanding process. Those of us who choose to mentor others must continue our own consultation where we discuss our conflicts, struggles, and confusions and have a safe place for our need to vent without fear of judgment. As experienced clinicians, we are responsible for bringing our best selves to our mentees; this requires that we also continue to be mentored. The support of our fellow clinicians is an invaluable gift of comfort and sustenance in the work we do. No matter how many years we have under our belts as clinicians, we never stop needing honest feedback and constructive criticism in the service of maintaining our professional integrity.

Mentorship is about passing the torch to the younger generation. It's a live process of guiding another person in ways that help them find themselves. To mentor is a commitment of time and energy and sharing competencies, interests, experience, and knowledge with another. It cannot be stressed enough that it is essential that the relationship between mentor and mentee be a fit for both people. You must be genuinely interested in your mentee as an individual. In the best of circumstances, the possibilities that occur in a mentor–mentee relationship are infinite and extend far beyond the time when the relationship existed. My mentor, James F. T. Bugental, died in 2008 and still remains in the consulting room with me.

In an article published on LinkedIn on thoughtfulness, Subir Chowdhury told stories of care and concern, writing: "Those moments are opportunities to act in a thoughtful way: to be attentive to others, considerate, unselfish, and provide comfort or aid."[10]

Being thoughtful requires that we listen to one another, that we pay attention on multiple levels to what another person is saying, and that we listen to ourselves and respond as authentically as possible. The capacity to be thoughtful entails bringing care to the people we are with, caring about what matters to us in our lives, and, ultimately, caring enough about ourselves that we pay attention to our inner world and what it is communicating with us. Integrating thoughtfulness into our work relationships helps us to feel that someone is there for us. We feel free to talk about whatever is on our mind and express feelings from our heart without fearing that we'll be judged or deemed inadequate for our vulnerabilities. Relationships based on this level of trust validate and encourage our common struggle to be human.

We need to advocate for one another and carve out time to develop our collegial relationships in our work. The camaraderie that is created when we value our need for connection with one another fills up the empty spaces of aloneness and isolation. We join each other in the trenches to help one another survive the battles, thrive in the meaningful moments of our work, and create clinical environments of camaraderie.

We engage every day in a serious line of work, and we are constantly dealing with consequential decisions and actions. Yes, it's important to be conscious, mindful, and thoughtful, but it's also important to have some fun with one another. Some of the best times I've had with other clinicians have involved shared activities of little to no consequence. It may be a cliché to say that laughter is the best medicine, but nowhere is this truer than in clinical work. Bonding through having goofy times together is a great relief from the sober and responsible nature of much of our work. Connecting in the lighter moments of our lives is the best thing we have for sticking together.

Trust that meaningful conversations, thoughtful words and gestures, and coming together in lighthearted play can change your world. We are drawn together when we listen to other people's stories, and it becomes hard to judge or fear a person whose story you know. Believe that we can depend on one another, that we are not adversaries but allies. Remember that we are all human and trust in the essential quality of human goodness. As Margaret Mead said: "Never doubt that a small group of thoughtful, committed citizens can change the world; indeed, it's the only thing that ever has."[11]

We don't need to continue to define and experience our clinical environment as a battlefield. Collaboration is the essence of life; our connection to one another as human beings is undeniable, and our success depends on all of us knowing and acting on this kinship. Stay together.

In regard to collaboration between clinicians, it takes a village to provide the best care.

—Dr. Jon Greif, email, July 20, 2016

Put down the weight of your aloneness and ease into the conversation.

—David Whyte, *Everything Is Waiting for You*[12]

This workbook section provides thoughts, suggestions, and resources for ways to build collaborative relationships with your fellow clinicians. The questions presented for your consideration invite you to begin a conversation within yourself, and with your colleagues, that helps to build a community you can rely on in the work that you do. Most of you have arrived at your work as a clinician because you answered a call to commit to the healing profession, so coming together as a group joins the strength of those individual commitments and serves all of you.

Find the courage to start a conversation that matters. Open up to people you know. Open up to people you don't know. Be brave and talk to people you have never approached and be curious about what you discover in these dialogues. Invite others to participate in discussing what's possible for the creation of meaningful work relationships. Collaboration is about enhancing each other's work and creating harmony, a way of being flexible and open with others. You can use this next section to identify your thoughts and feelings and to personalize your wants and needs for building camaraderie with your colleagues.

Identifying What Collaboration Means to You

- Write an in-depth definition of what you are looking for in your collegial relationships.

_____

_____

_____

_____

- Reflect on what you believe to be possible in regard to building collaborative collegial relationships. Write about the thoughts, feelings, images, and dreams that emerge for you in this exploration.

_____

_____

_____

_____

- What do you say and do to invite compassionate interaction with your colleagues?

_____

_____

_____

_____

- How would you like to be approached by others? Are you open and do you recognize when someone is extending themselves to you?

_____

_____

_____

_____

- How do you offer support, understanding, encouragement, or help to others?

_____

_____

_____

_____

- How would you like to be supported? What helps you feel understood and encouraged?

_____

_____

- What do you give in your work relationships?

_____

_____

_____

_____

- What won't you give?

_____

_____

_____

_____

- How do you create distance or push people away in your work environment? Are you conscious of when you do this?

_____

_____

_____

_____

- How do you negotiate relationships with difficult people at work?

_____

_____

_____

_____

- How do you bring your full presence into your work relationships?

_____

_____

_____

_____

How much do you allow yourself to show up with people you work with? Are you comfortable letting colleagues know you beyond your clinical role?

_____

_____

_____

_____

How do you play with your colleagues? What kinds of activities, events, or get-togethers would help you to have more fun and feel more connected with other clinicians?

_____

_____

_____

_____

Who do you turn to when you need support and understanding, encouragement, or help in your work? List the people you count as your allies at work. You may also want to think about people with whom you would like to form alliances.

_____

_____

_____

_____

Practices That Help Build Collaborative Partnerships

- Setting the intention to look for the best in others is one way to create collaborative work partnerships. When we greet another person with an open heart, they are likely to respond to us in kind. Choose to see the best in those around you and connect with them from your own best place.
- Practicing generosity with your colleagues opens warm connections. Sometimes just a smile or an encouraging text message can brighten up the day. A silly little gift can touch someone and make a difference

in their life. Show people small acts of kindness and sometimes stretch yourself to offer moments of generosity to people with whom you feel in conflict.

- Show appreciation to people on a consistent basis. Rather than coming from a negative focus on what others are not doing, concentrate and remark on what they are doing that you appreciate. Extend appreciation to people for who they are, not just for the tasks they perform. A simple acknowledgment conveys a caring message and lets others know that you see them as another human being. Say thank you often and acknowledge others frequently.

- Give someone a hug. It's often best to ask first so that your intentions are clear and people don't feel intruded on. We work in cerebral environments where we are always "too busy," so at times human touch is a reminder of how we all need personal contact.

- Finding a common and compassionate language helps us gain a sense of identity and the feeling of belonging to a community. Sometimes, you can develop phrases or lines from the experiences you have together. It helps for people to feel known and seen when we are speaking in words we understand. Remember to pay attention to how well you listen to what others are saying and respond to their words before moving on to what you have to say.

- Pay attention to nonverbal communication and all that happens in between the spoken lines of our conversations. Bringing curiosity to this level of communication helps develop a deeper sense of contact and understanding with others.

- Connecting with difficult people is one of the biggest challenges in our work as clinicians. We cannot change or control another person, so how successfully we approach edgy situations depends on the attitude we bring with us to the interaction. All of the suggestions covered so far in this workbook section are especially applicable when you are dealing with difficult and frustrating interactions with other clinicians. We can usually find some way to connect with another person regardless of our differences.

- Inviting others to join you and joining others when they invite you opens up numerous possibilities for bonding together as you work together. This can be as complicated as forming work groups or as simple as spending a few moments having a cup of coffee with a colleague. It involves taking the risk to ask others to join with you in your endeavors.

- Having fun with one another is without doubt the best of all worlds to foster meaningful connections, especially when most of our time is spent in highly responsible and often stressful situations. There is always time to have levity and hilarity in the midst of our busy days. And, depending on your personal choices, you can spend enjoyable time with your colleagues outside of work.

Structures That Help to Build Collaborative Partnership

Five guys on the court working together can achieve more than five talented individuals who come and go as individuals.

—Kareem Abdul-Jabbar[13]

- Form work groups for professional and personal support in order to share diverse perspectives, give and receive constructive feedback, develop communication skills, and build camaraderie among peers. These may be formal groups with facilitation, peer-led groups, or a combination of both. However, it is vital that these groups be regularly scheduled and attended in order for them to effectively address collegial collaboration. One to two meetings a month is optimal in order to create a group that provides a creative and safe outlet for expression.
- Establish work partnerships between other clinicians with a shared purpose and a common vision that builds trust and openness and recognizes the value and contribution of each person involved. Partnerships that are alive and grow will include shared goals and aims as well as the experience of feeling accepted and understood. They also promote an atmosphere of self-awareness and learning. In the spirit of openness and collaboration, partnerships offer the opportunity to facilitate a warm, humane work environment.
- Plan and create retreats that offer a time to get away with one another in an environment that is separate from the workplace. These can vary in length from a day to a weekend to a week, depending on what is possible within the framework of time and financial necessity. Retreats should not be totally focused on work tasks and

responsibilities, but rather include time for personal sharing, finding creative outlets, and having some enjoyable fun with each other. The intention is to build connections and bond in a more intimate way to support relationships at work. Settings outside of work, such as a retreat center in a natural setting, are ideal, but if this is not possible, even just going outside the usual structure and sitting outside can be conducive to the feeling of being on a retreat away from the normal day-to-day setting.

- Rely on online connections, such as chat groups or supportive listservs, that allow for a forum of discussion and which include private messaging. This way of building collaboration across the miles can be surprisingly satisfying as well as easy to access during a busy day or at home in the evening. Finding and joining an online group that feels collegial can serve as an ongoing resource of support and helps to cultivate collaborative relationships that have the potential to solidify over time.

- Build brief regular check-ins into your workday. This could be as simple as just saying "Hi, how are you?" in the hall or in someone's office. Five-minute check-ins with other clinicians can be done on the fly by asking someone if they have a moment to talk. More formalized time can be structured in order to prioritize the quality of the relationships at work and help to solidify a routine of paying attention to one another. It is also helpful to notice when a colleague appears harried or stressed and then asking how they are in that moment.

The Value of Collaboration

The feeling of belonging to a group is an essential human need and must be highlighted as a requisite condition in our work. Collaborative relationships in work contribute to personal satisfaction and create a sense of being part of the whole group and not just an isolated individual. Meaningful connections add to the well-being of all concerned and in that way fill the working environment with an atmosphere of cohesiveness, trust, care, and personal responsibility.

We spend numerous hours each week working with other clinicians, sometimes more time than we spend with our families and friends, so ensuring that the quality of that time is as high as possible is vital. It is our responsibility to ourselves and to those with whom we work. Our collaborative work partners are the friends who carry us through the bad times and celebrate with us as we sail through the good moments. They are the lifelong companions in this work, alongside us in the trenches. We take care of ourselves when we form meaningful relationships with other clinicians; by creating a community of support, we can help heal the difficulties of isolation and burnout for each one of us.

A friend is, as it were, a second self.

—Cicero[14]

Notes

1. Desert Fathers, in *Stories of the Spirit, Stories of the Heart: Parables of the Spiritual Path from Around the World*, edited by Christina Feldman and Jack Kornfield, Harper, San Francisco, 1991, p. 169. Excerpt from *Desert Wisdom* by Yushi Nomura, reprinted with permission from Orbis Books, New York, 2001, p. 17.

2. Michelle O'Daniel and Alan H. Rosenstein, Professional Communication and Team Collaboration, in *Patient Safety and Quality: An Evidence-Based Handbook for Nurses*, edited by Pamela G. Hughes, Agency for Healthcare Research and Quality, Rockville, MD, 2008, Chapter 33, p. 2.https://www.ncbi.nlm.nih.gov/books/NBK2637/. Reprinted with permission of the Agency for Healthcare Research and Quality.

3. O'Daniel and Rosenstein, Professional Communication.

4. O'Daniel and Rosenstein, Professional Communication.

5. Charles Darwin, Quotable Quote, Good reads. n.d. https://www.goodreads.com/quotes/368727-in-the-long-history-of-humankind-and-animal-kind-too.

6. Bill Withers, Lean on Me, from the record album *Still Bill*, Sussex Records, released April 21, 1972. Words and Music by Bill Withers, Reprinted by Permission of Hal Leonard, LLC.

7. Kathleen M. Sutcliffe, PhD, Elizabeth Lewton, PhD, MPH, and Marilynn M. Rosenthal, PhD, Communication Failures: An Insidious Contributor to Medical Mishaps. *Acad Med*. 2004;79(2):192.

8. J. R. R. Tolkien, *The Silmarillion*, edited and published posthumously by Christopher Tolkien, Allen and Unwin, London, September 15, 1977.

https://www.goodreads.com/quotes/518504-all-have-their-worth-and-each-contributes-to-the-worth

9. Harvard T. H. Chan School of Public Health, Who Mentored You: Maya Angelou. https://sites.sph.harvard.edu/wmy/celebrities/maya-angelou. Used with permission by Caged Bird Legacy, LLC.

10. Subir Chowdhury, The Power of a Glass of Water: Why Simple Acts of Thoughtfulness Matter Today. Linked In. https://www.linkedin.com/pulse/power-glass-water-why-simple-acts-thoughtfulness-matter-chowdhury. Published March 4, 2017.

11. Margaret Mead, Margaret Mead Quotes. BrainyQuote. n.d. https://www.brainyquote.com/quotes/quotes/m/margaretme100502.html.

12. David Whyte, *Everything Is Waiting for You*, Many Rivers Press, Langley, WA, 2003. http://www.davidwhyte.com/english-poetry/#Everything.

13. Kareem Abdul-Jabbar, Kareem Abdul-Jabbar Quotes. BrainyQuote. n.d. https://www.brainyquote.com/quotes/kareem_abduljabbar_370629.

14. Marcus Tullius Cicero, Marcus Tullius Cicero Quote. BrainyQuote. n.d. https://www.brainyquote.com/quotes/marcus_tullius_cicero_156345.

CHAPTER 8

Personal Narrative in Survivorship Care

Telling Your Story

Tell me the facts and I'll learn.
Tell me the truth and I'll believe.
But tell me a story
And it will live
In my heart forever

—Native American proverb[1]

You have a story of your work and the calling that brought you to it. It's a story that wants to be told, a story that only you can tell. In fact, you are filled with stories of the hours, days, months, and years of your educational experiences, the beginnings of your work life and eventually your ongoing career serving patients and their families who are dealing with numerous types of cancer diagnoses. As cancer screening and treatment improves, many of these people are moving forward into cancer survivorship, which, while fantastic, comes with both physical and emotional complications and complexities.

My book *Surviving the Storm: A Workbook for Telling Your Cancer Story* provides a narrative structure for cancer patients and their communities to tell the story of their cancer experience as a way to deepen their healing. In lieu of supporting clinicians in person-centered care, this section of *Psychosocial Care of Cancer Survivors* is designed to give you a narrative structure to tell your story. Patient stories tell you about who they are; your story expresses who you are. Sharing your story introduces you in a holistic manner that acknowledges you as a whole person, not just the clinical role that you inhabit. Exploring and knowing your own story leads you to an understanding of yourself, a deeper knowing of who you are and how you came to where you are now. It's like weaving together the threads of your past into a continuous cloth. Telling your story connects you with others. These intimate tales bring us closer to our own humanness and remind us of our identity as healers. We remember that we are all human beings and that we are in this together. In an interview in *The Sun Magazine*, Raymond Barr, MD, said, "Medicine is all story. It is dense with story."[2]

A narrative approach in person-centered care is valuable not only for the patients but also for the clinicians, as it provides a way to humanize personal and professional experience in a dehumanizing healthcare system. Storytelling is the most ancient form of communication. Stories told through the spoken word existed prior to the written word, the printed page, the computer, and Twitter. Throughout the ages, stories have remained an essential human way to connect with one another and express who we are, and the more difficult the narrative, the more essential it is for our stories to be told and for us to be heard. Sharing our stories joins us together when we feel like everything around us seems to have crashed and burned. Stories are an outstretched hand when we are suffering, and they become a high five in our moments of elation. In these narrations, we offer both ourselves and the accumulated knowledge that we gain through our own experiences.

Knowledge can be shared in numerous ways; indeed, we live in a world where we are constantly bombarded with facts and information. In our current media environment, we need a healthy dose of skepticism regarding reports, studies, and innovations that may or not be accurate or helpful. Our psyches are struggling to take in the amount of information that is thrown at us and we feel buried in data that we struggle to keep track of, much less remember. However, most of us remember people, our experiences, and even facts when we listen to a personal story. Telling someone about your experience breathes life into the interaction and changes the dulled experience of being lectured into an animated and genuine moment of communication. This may be because when we are touched by stories we can identify with, they give us the chance to reflect on ourselves, our own experiences, and remind us that there is always the possibility of transformation.

We create new stories as our lives change, as we continue to have new and different experiences, and as our work grows and matures, so it is natural that we will continually have new stories to tell. Telling our stories is not the same as being attached to a personal story, or myth, that you carry as a definition of who you are as a person. It's not about staying stuck in an image of yourself that no longer fits who you are. Being with your stories in an authentic way is a fluid, growing experience of connecting, reflecting, and expressing yourself in the present moment in a narrative form.

Stories Shared by Clinicians

Some of the stories that follow come from my own interviews with clinicians who I spoke with in person. Some of them are responses to written material that I sent out broadly in the form of a questionnaire. I made numerous attempts to interview other clinicians and was always greeted with enthusiastic interest. I heard brief comments from them about their distress and their thoughts, validating the importance of clinicians having a place to voice their stories. However, in the end, the majority of the clinicians I approached didn't reply to the narrative questions on the questionnaire. This seemed to me to parallel the difficulties this community has in regard to creating personal space and time in their lives, as well as giving themselves the permission to find ways to reflect and time for reflection. I have included personal interviews I was able to obtain in this chapter, as well as stories I found written by clinicians in various other sources, such as blogs, articles, websites, and elsewhere.

Cheryl Krauter, MFT

This short version of the story of how I came to the choice of becoming a psychotherapist and what led me to work in cancer healthcare is an example of how we can find ourselves following surprising paths that we could never have imagined for ourselves.

My own story as a psychotherapist begins in 1968 when, as a 17-year-old college freshman, I was introduced to encounter groups and experimental psychotherapies. Although I would not begin my formal education and training until 1976, I entered a path of awareness and consciousness in those early, sometimes "wild, wild, West" days of psychology in the late 1960s. In 1977, I found a book in my university library called *The Search for Authenticity* by James F. T. Bugental (New York: Holt, Rinehart, and Winston, 1965) and, after years of experimentation and a deep dissatisfaction with behavioral methods and psychological frameworks based on pathology, I found a home in existential humanistic therapy, which became the foundation for my work as a psychotherapist.

Fast-forward to 2007 when I was diagnosed with metastatic triple-negative breast cancer and endured a grueling treatment; I remain to this day in remission. I am fortunate to be a cancer survivor. However, I noticed a definite lack of attention and services for survivors who wanted to explore the physical and emotional trauma of their experiences with a cancer diagnosis as well as the difficult waters that awaited them in the post-treatment period. I was extremely ambivalent about working in the world of cancer, partially due to the reality that I would need to reenter, negotiate, and cope with the medical model of practice that I had removed myself from years ago.

I wondered how it would be for me to sit with people who were dealing with the issues of cancer. Would I be constantly triggered and fearful myself as I listened to their concerns? I worried that I might be overwhelmed by the horrific and terrifying storms that wreak havoc when you receive the news: "You have cancer." And I knew, without a doubt, that I would have to stand tall and demand to be taken seriously by other professionals who would not consider my humanistic, contemplative background valid in an evidenced-based healthcare system. In the end, I chose to stay, face forward, and walk into cancer healthcare because I believe that there is a need for attention to humanistic survivorship care. I call my work with cancer "the specialty that chose me," and I have never regretted taking that call when it came.

Raymond Barfield, MD (Excerpted from *The Sun*)

I was touched by this story and include it because it shows kindness in the face of terror and grief, a capacity to listen to the needs of a parent losing a child and the willingness to provide the possibility of grace in profound loss.

A mentor of mine, a pediatric professor at Emory, had a three-year old son with metastatic neuroblastoma. The cancer was everywhere. I was the little boy's doctor in the intensive care unit (ICU) night after night. I watched my mentor go from being a professor to being a terrified mother. She began to suggest improbable treatments to me: Couldn't I do granulocyte transfusions or something? She was desperate to save her son, who was hooked up to IV drips, overmedicated, completely unhappy, unable to sleep, and experiencing chronic fatigue, on top of being a very sick three-year-old. We all knew he was dying.

One day, my mentor was lying next to her son in the ICU bed where he was miserable, and she just looked at me and said, "We're going home." I was floored, but I did everything that was needed to be done to release him, and my mentor and her husband brought their little boy home to their own bed, where they lay together for a few more days before he died surrounded by his family.[3]

Robert Pearl, MD (Excerpted from KevinMD.com)

This story reminds me of all that we can learn from our patients; it addresses this doctor's courageous openness not only to his patient, but also to his own vulnerability.

Shortly after the birth of his son, I had to give Paul the sad news that his cancer had spread to his lung. I explained that chemotherapy would slow its progression, but a cure was not possible. As he had done with everything about his disease, he understood and accepted the facts and the implications. For the next several months, his oncologist provided most of his care, so I rarely saw him as a patient. But, he always sought me out and updated me on his life and his family. We shared an interest in growing fruits and vegetables in our yards, and invariably, he would bring me a juicy tomato or a peach.

I was saddened to watch as the tumor spread and his condition worsened. One day, he came to my office and asked to talk. He had brought with him a present for me: a self-portrait he had sketched with charcoals. On the back he had written, "Life ends and we should enjoy each day." And in his joking style, he added, "You will never be a good farmer, but if you work hard at it, you might become a great physician."

He concluded, "Please do this for your patients and for me."

With tears in my eyes, I hugged him and thanked him for the beautiful picture and the inspiration. Sometimes the most difficult part of being a physician—and the most important—is accepting our limitations and letting go.[4]

Erin Barnes (Excerpted from statnews.com)

I offer this story as an illustration of the difficulties that students experience in their rigorous education and training. It shows a level of condescension that is all too familiar in the hierarchical healthcare system and presents a classic and frightening portrait of burnout.

The hold music on the telephone cut off abruptly as the doctor I was trying to reach picked up the line. "Yes?" she said curtly.

"Hi, this is Erin Barnes," I said. She then goes on to describe the patient issue.

"I'm sorry," the doctor interrupted, "who is this I am speaking with?" I felt my face start to flush.

"Is this a resident?" she asked. I could hear the anger in her voice.

"I . . . no, I'm a sub-intern."

"You have got to be kidding me," the doctor continued, "A student? You're a student calling me? Wow." I held the phone away from my ear, as it if would somehow protect me from her verbal assault.

She was just warming up.

I don't remember how the conversation ended. I just remember that when it finally did, I was struck with the horrifying thought: What if I end up like her?

The doctor was once a student like me. Now she is using vulgar language to describe a patient and flying into a rage because a sub-intern called her. The interaction shook me, mostly because I knew I wasn't immune to becoming a doctor like her.[5]

Merideth Shamszad, MFT, Private Practice (Written Interview)

This private practice psychotherapist speaks to the difficulties of finding ways to coordinate and collaborate with other professionals that are all too common in the vast healthcare system. Her story highlights the distressing and familiar barriers to communication between clinicians.

In private practice I am limited by time, confidentiality constraints, distance, and resources. I do not feel able to establish collaboration with other caregivers regarding my clients, and it doesn't feel good! I am even thinking about developing a different informed consent form for my clients with illness that will give me permission to talk to others on their care team. For example, I recently lost a client to cancer. For a week or two before she died she was in a lot of pain and it was not being managed well. I wanted to call her doctor or her case manager, but never had a chance to get releases, as her illness progressed very quickly at that point.

Cassandra Falby, MFT, Program Director, Women's Cancer Resource Center (In-Person Interview)

This poignant story is from a clinician who works in the community; it brings home the often-heartbreaking difficulties of providing care in the underserved communities and the impact on the clinicians who navigate through them.

I've worked with people who have cancer and are living in their cars or in homeless shelters while they are in treatment. I was helping one woman pack up what few possessions she had so that she could go and be with her sister but she died before she could get there. I'm with the people who are in a relationship with cancer patients who will deeply, deeply miss their partners, parents, children, and it breaks my heart. Coming in every day, helping clients, and offering alternatives helps my heart.

Rafael Campo, MD (Online Story)

I found this beautiful tale that reminds us that the patients we are caring for are not statistics and how important it is to allow ourselves to be present and give attention to the people we are sitting with in their illnesses.

When I visited my grandmother in the hospital in the last weeks before she died, I cried for a while into her shoulder. But by then I was a young doctor, so soon I headed for the nurses' station and pored over her hospital chart while she lay propped up in her bed, the glass and metal ICU like the internal workings of some incomprehensible machine designed for time travel. Countless hours and hundreds of thousands of dollars had gone into the attempt to transform me from a long-term financial burden on my parents to someone with a respectable, money-making career. She was in heart failure despite being on dialysis, and I tried desperately to understand her fluid imbalances. Her I's and O's were dutifully tabulated, in a sequence that suggested a code whose rules I might decipher. In my exasperation, I looked up from the record of her gradual demise, and caught a glimpse of her as she fingered her rosary, praying to herself with a peaceful smile on her face, taking her own measure of her receding life. When I write about her now, all the data that seemed so important then have faded to insignificance—but it is that one cherished detail in my memory, this one little story, that always makes her come alive to me again.[6]

Storytelling Clinicians

There is a growing movement to support creativity in healthcare. More clinicians are writing about their experiences and speaking up about the need for the future of healthcare to move in a more holistic direction, which includes and integrates the arts, focuses on inventive ways of providing services, and encourages an overall willingness to allow thinking outside of the box as a way to refresh a stale system. The need to humanize our work shows up in the call to return to the art of medicine and the creation of a more personal connection with the work that we do. The individuals and groups in the list that follows are prime examples of those who have created ways to address the importance of narrative. I include them as people who have inspired and encouraged me to continue to confront an impersonal system. As clinicians, we all owe a debt of gratitude to those who risk standing up and making themselves heard in regard to the need for humanizing healthcare.

- Abraham Verghese, MD, physician and writer, in his 2014 TEDMD talk, spoke about a "lack of metaphor" in healthcare and how this failure of imagination has affected the current disengaged healthcare system. You can listen to his talk on metaphor at http://www.tedmed.com/talks/show?id=292979.
- The Nocturnists is a group of healthcare professionals in San Francisco who write and sometimes perform the stories of their work. Founded by Dr. Emily Silverman when she was a second-year resident in internal medicine at the University of California San Francisco, their mission statement, on The Nocturnists' website

(http://thenocturnists.com) states: "We collect and share stories about the physician experience because: 1. People want to hear them. . . . 2. It's therapeutic. . . . 3. It's important. . . . 4. It's fun!" Silverman told the *San Francisco Chronicle* in an interview (May 18, 2016), "As an internist, there are so many things that happen to me that I don't even remember. It's just like boom, boom—one emergency after the next. I wish I had written some of it down. There are so many stories that went untold and unprocessed. This is a good way to do that."[7]

- The Doctors Who Create website (http://www.doctorswhocreate. com) states: "We want to change the culture of medicine to encourage and reward creativity. We're starting by highlighting creative things that are already happening, cultivating physician and student networks, and providing inspiration for future physicians. In the future, we hope to arrange conferences, contests, and scholarships for creative people in medicine."[8]

- KevinMD.com (http://www.kevinmd.com/blog), an online journal founded in 2004 by Kevin Pho, MD, features stories and articles written by clinicians on a multitude of topics that are often taboo in the traditional medical setting. I receive regular updates from this site and refer to it on an ongoing basis as a way to be informed about the personal struggles that those in healthcare bear as well as to read the stories clinicians share. The site not only provides useful information, but also gives clinicians a forum to express themselves in order to break their silence and let their voices be heard. The KevinMD website states: "Thousands of authors contribute to KevinMD.com: front-line primary care doctors, surgeons, specialist physicians, nurses, medical students, policy experts. And of course, patients, who need the medical profession to hear their voices."[9]

Listening to Stories: It's Not Just About Telling

When someone really listens to us, our blood flows in his or her veins. That person is moved as we are by our history, passions, hurts, binds, values, joys: in short, by the integrity of our existence.

—Carl A. Faber, *On Listening*[10]

The other side of the power of telling your story is the power of listening to the stories of others. Eager to express ourselves, we sometimes perch on the edge of our seats, waiting for a pause in the conversation to tell our stories rather than being still and listening to the person who is telling us their story. We can fall prey to this with colleagues, patients, our partners, and so on. But, when we don't listen, not only do we miss the opportunity to know someone else, but also we lose the chance to learn something about ourselves in relationship. Listening to someone's story can be a very moving experience that touches our own hearts and gives us insight not only into the storyteller but also into ourselves.

When you listen to someone's story, pay attention to the silence, the pause between words, the downward glance, the sighs. Listening is not only auditory but also visual. Listening is about bringing your presence to the conversation and giving attention to another person as they tell their story. This is the moment where we are told to silence our phones, shut down our computers, look up, and open our hearts to someone who is telling us their story. Sometimes, we just need to shut up and listen.

The workbook section of this chapter offers a structure for you to reflect within yourself and recall your own story. Take the time to listen to the voice within you as you reflect on the questions and notice what emerges as you go deeper into yourself. You may return periodically to this section to update it, expand it, or add to your stories. It's up to you to decide how you will share your story. There are times when we need to stay in a place of contemplation, when it's important to remain within ourselves for a while, and at other times we are bursting to tell our stories. Then, it is important to choose who will hear your story. There are no hard-and-fast rules in this exploration except for you to allow yourself to honor your own story.

You have a story to tell. What is it?

Part I: Suggestions on How to Write Your Story

- Use the space provided in this book to write your story.
- Get a special journal to create the book of your story.
- Create a file on your computer that is specifically for your story.
- Create a timeline on paper or on your computer. Mark dates starting with your decision to become a clinician and continue on to the present time. Match events with the emotional experiences that occurred for you.
- Plan a personal retreat to write your story.

Part II: Prompts to Help You Tell Your Story

- Start from the beginning and remember when you decided to become a clinician.
- Go back to your first memories of this choice and then bring yourself up to present time.
- Reflect on significant events and periods of time.
- Bring to mind individuals and groups who are important to your story.

- As best as you can, recall the thoughts and feelings associated with these experiences.
- Start from where you are now and work backward to the beginning of your work life.

Part III: Questions to Help You Tell Your Story

- When did I first know that I wanted to be a healthcare clinician?

_____

_____

_____

_____

- How did I imagine myself as a clinician? What intentions and goals did I begin with when I began my education?

_____

_____

_____

_____

- What were my hopes and dreams at the beginning of my journey?

_____

_____

_____

_____

- How do I define myself as a clinician?

_____

_____

_____

_____

- How do I see myself now as a clinician? Have I satisfied my intentions? Have I reached my goals?

_____

_____

_____

_____

- What have I been told about myself as a clinician? How do people see me?

_____

_____

_____

_____

- What I tell myself about me . . .

_____

_____

_____

_____

- What I really know about me . . .

_____

_____

_____

_____

- What are five things that you appreciate about yourself as a clinician? Write them down. If more than five occur to you, write them down!

_____

_____

_____

_____

- How do I make a difference in the lives of others?

_____

_____

_____

_____

- Who has inspired me in my work and in my life? What was it that touched me?

_____

_____

_____

_____

- Describe the relationship between your inner self and the professional self you present to the world.

_____

_____

_____

_____

- Name and write about the challenges you feel proud of facing in your clinical work.

_____

_____

_____

_____

- What are the challenges that you currently face in your work?

_____

_____

_____

_____

- Can you remember a time in your life when you felt alone?

_____

_____

_____

_____

- Is there an achievement or contribution that you are most proud of? Why?

_____

_____

_____

_____

- I have learned that . . .

_____

_____

_____

_____

- What has been most surprising to you in your work?

_____

_____

_____

_____

- What do you most regret having not done? What can you learn from this as you move forward?

_____

_____

_____

_____

- What particular moments or memories in your work stand out for you?

_____

_____

_____

_____

- As a clinician, I have been changed by . . .

_____

_____

_____

_____

- Imagining your clinical work years into the future, what do you see?

_____

_____

_____

_____

- What are your hopes and dreams as you continue your journey as a clinician?

_____

_____

_____

_____

- How would you like to be remembered?

_____

_____

_____

_____

Part IV: Tell Your Story

It all began when . . .

Tell Your Story (continued)

Notes

1. Native American Proverb.
2. Raymond Barr, MD, The Miracle in Front of You. *The Sun Magazine*, January 2016, p. 15.
3. Barr, Miracle, p. 6.
4. Robert Pearl, MD, How Our Patients Make Us Better. KevinMD.com. https://www.kevinmd.com/blog/2016/06/patients-make-us-better.html. Published June 19, 2016, p. 3.
5. Erin Barnes, To Fight Physician Burnout, I'm Making a Binder of Medical Successes. *STAT*. https://www.statnews.com/2017/04/05/physician-burnout-document-medical-success/. Published April 5, 2017, p. 2.
6. Rafael Campo, MD, Illness as Muse. *Bellevue Literary Rev*. Fall 2011. http://blr.med.nyu.edu/content/current/illnessasmuse.
7. Beth Spotswood, Doctors' Storytelling Evening the Right Kind of Medicine. *San Francisco Chronicle*, May 18, 2016. http://www.sfchronicle.com/entertainment/article/Doctors-storytelling-evening-the-right-kind-of-7644051.php.
8. Doctors Who Create. Home page. http://www.doctorswhocreate.com.
9. Kevin Pho, MD, About KevinMD.com. https://www.kevinmd.com/blog/about-kevin-md. Accessed January 12, 2018.
10. Carl A. Faber, *On Listening*, Perseus Press, New York, 1976, p. 3.

A Short History of Medicine
2000 bc: "Here, eat this root."
1000 bc: "That root is heathen, say this prayer."
1850 ad: "That prayer is superstition, drink this potion."
1940 ad: "That potion is snake oil, swallow this pill."
1985 ad: "That pill is ineffective, take this antibiotic."
2000 ad: "That antibiotic is artificial. Here, eat this root."

—Author unknown

In the years since 2007 when I was diagnosed with cancer, I have become aware of the profound complexities of the disease known as cancer. Once I entered the world of psychosocial oncology as a psychotherapist, I began to learn firsthand about the many twists, turns, and potholes in the highways and byways of the cancer healthcare system. As a clinician who is a cancer survivor, I live in both the world of the provider and the world of the patient, and this has given me the capacity to understand the perspectives of both groups. As a cancer survivor, I bring personal knowledge of the experience of cancer to my work with those who are dealing with a diagnosis of cancer. Many patients feel joined, understood, and less alone when they speak with someone who has also been down that rough road of cancer.

Working as a clinician in private practice makes me an outlier in my travels through cancer healthcare and in this way has given me the opportunity to be in the position of an outside observer participating within the system. As I become more involved in cancer healthcare, I have been able to bring depth psychotherapeutic work into the existing system as well as to learn from the clinicians providing services to cancer survivors who work within that system. Our work together has grown and developed, validating the strong potential possible in collaborative endeavors between clinicians.

Over the years, my compassion and respect for the clinicians who work within cancer healthcare has grown, and I have deep empathy for the arduous, complicated, and frustrating issues they face on a daily basis. The conflicts involved in providing person-centered care to patients and the essential need for attention to the well-being of clinicians are widespread and serious. Within healthcare, we have moved too far from our human need for relationship, both with our patients, our colleagues, and, most important, with ourselves. Edwin Leap, MD, said it beautifully: "There was a time of collegiality. There was a time when we discussed cases and our feelings and our sorrow and our passion. That was when medicine was about people."[1] In essence, we have come full circle to the importance of the human relationship as it relates to the multiple layers of healing involved in cancer survivorship care.

The National Institutes of Health's Office of Cancer Survivorship reported that as of January 2016 there were an estimated 15.5 million cancer survivors in the United States, and that the number of cancer survivors is projected to increase by 31%, to 20.3 million, by 2026, which represents an increase of more than 4 million survivors in 10 years.[2] Statistics on the impact of cancer and the issues of survivorship in the global community have not been reported since 2012, making the statistics gathered at that time currently irrelevant.

In 2017, the *Journal of Clinical Oncology* published an update on survivorship care that stated: "The field has begun to realize that the real challenge in cancer survivorship is not just the development of the survivorship care plan tool, but the optimization of the survivorship care planning process in such a way as to result in more tailored and coordinated care and, ultimately, decreased rates of preventable morbidity and mortality after cancer." The article went on to assert that "best practices have to be disseminated and implemented in real-world settings."[3]

There are three vital points to glean from this statement:

- We need survivorship care plans that are more tailored to the individual.
- The importance of coordinated care in survivorship care cannot be understated.
- Best practices need to be disseminated and implemented in real-world settings.

The recognition and naming of these points in cancer survivorship is a call to action in response to the need for communication and coordination between survivors, clinicians, formal and informal caregivers, and all others who attend to the needs of those in post-treatment as well as those who are living with cancer. Both of my books, *Surviving the Storm: A Workbook for Telling Your Cancer Story* (Krauter, 2017) and this volume, highlight relevant education in person-centered care, present practical structures to assist clinicians, and offer pragmatic real-world suggestions, resources, and alternatives that address taking action to deal with individualized survivorship plans, coordinated care, and the dissemination and implementation of quality survivorship care.

However, no plan or mode of action will be successful without our wholehearted engagement as clinicians who are committed to bringing human, person-centered quality into our work. By accepting our own vulnerability, as well as the vulnerability of our patients and our colleagues, we will always return to a stance of kindness and compassion that will open our minds and our hearts and give us a way to create the kind of relationships that are optimal for healing.

Awareness and recognition of our own experiences and the experiences of others allows us to develop the capacity to respond in a genuine, authentic way that can transform how we are and who we are in our work. This perspective represents a fundamental shift in our priorities as clinicians as it focuses on our responsibility to ourselves and to our colleagues. We need to find the courage and the fortitude to make these fundamental changes and connect with the place within us that made a commitment to our work in the first place. It's time to come home.

Notes

1. Edwin Leap, MD, KevinMD, Hospital CEOs Please Listen to Your Doctors and Nurses, March 15, 2016. https://www.medpagetoday.com/blogs/kevinmd/56862. Updated October 17, 2016.
2. National Institute of Health, National Cancer Institute, Office of Cancer Survivorship. Statistics. https://cancercontrol.cancer.gov/ocs/statistics/statistics.html. Last updated October 17, 2016.
3. Larissa Nekhlyudov, Patricia A. Ganz, Neeraj K. Arora, and Julia H. Rowland, Going Beyond Being Lost in Transition: A Decade of Progress in Cancer Survivorship. *J Clin Oncol.* 2017;35(18):1978–1981. http://ascopubs.org/doi/full/10.1200/JCO.2016.72.1373.

Resources

Gathering resources for clinicians working in cancer healthcare has been a challenge as most of the resources for cancer survivorship are generally more focused on patient care than on the professional education, training, and personal well-being of clinicians working within the healthcare system. To have a better understanding of the challenges that clinicians face in dealing with the complex issues of survivorship, we need resources that broaden the knowledge of relevant cancer survivor issues, address the importance of psychosocial training for clinicians, target methods of clear communication, and develop workable modes of the dissemination of information while creating active referral systems.

Finding Local Resources

Resources in your local community can be of great value to both you and your patients. You can contact your local health department, community mental health agency, or family services agency as well as familiarize yourself with local cancer centers, especially those with the capacity to offer services free of charge. You can locate clinicians working in the community who specialize in working with cancer patients and their support systems by asking your colleagues for referrals and also checking on *Psychology Today*'s website (https://www.psychologytoday.com), which includes a therapist finder feature listed by specialties. One of the most valuable sources of information on local resources is networking with other clinicians as word of mouth is still one of the best ways to connect clinicians with one another. The following organizations can assist you in gathering local resources:

- American Cancer Society
  https://www.cancer.org/treatment/support-programs-and-services.html
- American Psychosocial Oncology Society (APOS)
  https://apos-society.org
- CancerCare

https://www.cancercare.org/publications/60-finding_resources_in_your_community
- Cancer Support Community
  https://www.cancersupportcommunity.org/resources
- International Psychosocial Oncology Society (IPOS)
  https://ipos-society.org
- National Cancer Survivorship Resource Center
  https://www.cancer.org/health-care-professionals/national-cancer-survivorship-resource-center.html

Resources for Personal and Professional Development

An ongoing personal commitment to your own well-being is the essential foundation for the practice of bringing a human perspective to your clinical work. In the words of the ancient sage Chuang Tzu, "The perfect man of old looked after himself first before looking to help others." Finding what is meaningful to you in your continued development as a clinician is, and should be, extremely personal to who you are as an individual. As discussed in this book, being a lifelong learner not only enhances your clinical work but also contributes to your personal well-being. Once we make the choice to step on the path of helping others, taking an oath of helping ourselves becomes of equal significance.

Chapters 6 and 7 of *Psychosocial Care of Cancer Survivors* were designed to help guide you in the process of self-care and collaborative relationships with other clinicians. You may refer to these chapters in terms of creating doable ways to attend to your needs as a clinician. It is clear that nothing replaces a personal commitment to personal and professional growth.

The short list that follows has reading material that can support your ongoing education, professional development, and personal enhancement.

Suggested Reading

Bugental, James F. T., PhD, *Psychotherapy and Process: The Fundamentals of an Existential-Humanistic Approach*, Addison-Wesley, Boston, 1978.
Bugental, James F. T., PhD, *The Search for Authenticity*, Irvington, New York, 1981.
Bugental, James F. T., PhD, *The Art of the Psychotherapist*, Norton, New York, 1987.

Children's Oncology Group Nursing Discipline Clinical Practice Subcommittee/ Survivorship in collaboration with the Late Effects Committee, Wendy Landier, editor, *Establishing and Enhancing Services for Childhood Cancer Survivors: Long-Term Follow-up Program Resource Guide*, Children's Oncology Group, Monrovia, CA, 2007.

Chodrun, Pema, *Living Beautifully with Uncertainty and Change*, Shambhala, Boston, 2012.

Faber, Carl A., PhD, *On Listening*, Perseus Press, New York, 1976.

Gawande, Atul, MD, *Being Mortal: Medicine and What Matters in the End*, Metropolitan Books, Holt, New York, 2014.

Kalanithi, Paul, *When Breath Becomes Air*, Random House, New York, 2016.

Kornfield, Jack, *The Wise Heart: A Guide to the Universal Teachings of Buddhist Psychology*, Bantam Dell, New York, 2008.

Krauter, Cheryl, *Surviving the Storm: A Workbook for Telling Your Cancer Story*, Oxford University Press, New York, 2017.

McCabe, M. S., Bhatia, S., Oeffinger, K. C., et al., American Society of Clinical Oncology Statement: Achieving High-Quality Cancer Survivorship Care. *J Clin Oncol.* 2013;31(5):631–640.

Mukherjee, Siddhartha, MD, *The Laws of Medicine: Field Notes from an Uncertain Science*, Ted Books, Simon and Schuster, New York, 2015.

Schneider, Kirk, J., and Krug, Orah, *Existential Humanistic Therapy*, American Psychological Association, Washington, DC, 2010.

Silver, J. K., Strategies to overcome cancer survivorship barriers. *PM R.* 2011;3(6):503–506.

Wallin, David J., PhD, *Attachment in Psychotherapy*, Guilford Press, New York, 2017.

Yalom, Irvin D., MD, *The Gift of Therapy*, HarperCollins, New York, 2002.

Bibliography

Abdul-Jabbar, Kareem, Kareem Abdul-Jabbar Quotes, BrainyQuote. n.d. https://www.brainyquote.com/quotes/kareem_abduljabbar_370629.

Adichie, Chimamanda Ngozi, The Danger of a Single Story [TED talk], presented at TEDGlobal 2009, July, Oxford, UK.

Amiel, Henri-Frederic, *The Journal Intime of Henri-Frederic Amiel,* Vol. 2, August 1883, translated by Mrs. Mary Humphrey Ward, Burt, New York, 1889.

Babauta, Leo, A Guide to Cultivating Compassion in Your Life, with 7 Practices. https://zenhabits.net/a-guide-to-cultivating-compassion-in-your-life-with-7-practices. Published June 4, 2007.

Barnes, Erin, To Fight Physician Burnout, I'm Making a Binder of Medical Successes, *STAT*. https://www.statnews.com/2017/04/05/physician-burnout-document-medical-success/. Published April 5, 2017.

Barr, Raymond MD, The Miracle in Front of You. *The Sun Magazine*, January 2016, pp. 6, 8, 15.

Beckett, Samuel, *Endgame*, Grove Press, New York, 1992; premiered April 3, 1957, Royal Court Theatre, London.

Birnbaum, Robert, Rafael Campo. *The Morning News*, January 2004, p. 7. https://themorningnews.org/article/birnbaum-v.-rafael-campo.

Boyle, Brian, A Patient's Advice on How to Improve the Health Care Experience, Kevin MD.com. https://www.kevinmd.com/blog/2016/11/patients-advice-improve-health-care-experience.html. Published November 7, 2016. From Brian Boyle, *The Patient Experience*, reprinted by permission of Skyhorse Publishing, Inc.

Bowman, John, Changing the World: Arts and Medicine, interview with Jack Coulehan, MD, The Institute for Poetic Medicine, Palo Alto, CA, n.d. http://www.poeticmedicine.org/jack-coulehan.html.

Brown, John, Sunbeams. *The Sun Magazine*, December 2014. http://thesunmagazine.org/issues/468/sunbeams.

Buchanan, Natasha, PhD, Alleviate Cancer Survivor Distress: Screening and Psychosocial Care. http://www.medscape.com/viewarticle/864507. Published June 20, 2016.

Bugental, James F. T., *Psychotherapy and Process: The Fundamentals of an Existential-Humanistic Approach*, Addison-Wesley, Boston, 1978.

Bugental, James F. T., *The Search for Authenticity*, Irvington, New York, 1981.

Bugental, James F. T., *The Art of the Psychotherapist*, Norton, New York, 1987.

Campo, Rafael, MD, Illness as Muse. *Bellevue Literary Rev.* Fall 2011. http://blr.med.nyu.edu/content/current/illnessasmuse.

Campo, Rafael, MD, Hospital Writing Workshop, copyright © 2014 by Rafael Campo. *Comfort Measures Only: New and Selected Poems 1994–2016*, Duke University Press, Durham, NC, April 2018. In Poem-A-Day, January 3, 2014. https://www.poets.org/poetsorg/poem-day.

Carver, Raymond, What the Doctor Said, in *All of Us: Collected Poems*, Harvill Press, London, 1996, p. 113. © Harvill Press, 1996.

Chen, Pauline W., MD, The Widespread Problem of Doctor Burnout. *New York Times*, August 23, 2012.

Chetty, Raj, PhD, Stepner, Michael, BA, Abraham, Sarah, BA, et al., The Association Between Income and Life Expectancy in the United States, 2001–2014. *JAMA.* 2016;315(16):1750–1766. doi:10.1001/jama.2016.

Chodrun, Pema, *Living Beautifully with Uncertainty and Change*, Shambhala, Boston, 2012.

Chowdhury, Subir, The Power of a Glass of Water: Why Simple Acts of Thoughtfulness Matter Today, LinkedIn. https://www.linkedin.com/pulse/power-glass-water-why-simple-acts-thoughtfulness-matter-chowdhury. Published March 4, 2017.

Cicero, Marcus Tullius, Marcus Tullius Cicero Quotes, BrainyQuote. n.d. https://www.brainyquote.com/quotes/marcus_tullius_cicero_156345.

Coulehan, Jack, MD, Take Off Your Clothes [Poetry and Medicine]. *JAMA*. 2016;315(6):615.

Darwin, Charles, Quotable Quote, Goodreads. n.d. https://www.goodreads.com/quotes/368727-in-the-long-history-of-humankind-and-animal-kind-too.

Dhand, Suneel, MD, We Need Fewer Doctor MBAs and More Doctor Healers, KevinMD.com. http://www.kevinmd.com/blog/2014/06/need-fewer-doctor-mbas-doctor-healers.html. Published June 20, 2014.

Doctors Who Create. Homepage. http://www.doctorswhocreate.com.

Doidge, Norman, Every Patient Has a Story Worth Hearing [Blog], *Stanford Medicine 25*. https://stanfordmedicine25.stanford.edu/blog/archive/2016/Every-Patient-Has-a-Story-Worth-Hearing.html. Published March 22, 2016.

Erikson, Joan Serson, interview with Daniel Goleman. *New York Times*, June 14, 1988. http://www.nytimes.com/books/99/08/22/specials/erikson-old.html.

Faber, Carl A., PhD, *On Listening*, Perseus Press, New York, 1976.

Frost, Robert, A Time to Talk, in *Mountain Interval*, Holt, New York, 1920, p. 44.

Gallagher, Nora, Sunbeams. *The Sun Magazine*, January 2016. http://thesunmagazine.org/issues/481/sunbeams.

Gawande, Atul, MD, Big Med [Annals of Health Care]. *The New Yorker*, August 13, 2012, p. 18.

Gawande, Atul, *Being Mortal: Medicine and What Matters in the End*, Metropolitan Books, Holt, New York, 2014.

Goldberg, Carey, Harvard Study: Elderly Hospital Patients Live Longer, Do Better with Female Doctors. *CommonHealth*. December 19, 2016. http://www.wbur.org/commonhealth/2016/12/19/harvard-female-physicians-outcomes.

Goodman, Sandra G., How to Teach Doctors Empathy. *The Atlantic*, March 15, 2015.

Grumet, Jordan, MD, Assure Patients That We Are on Their Side. KevinMD. http://www.kevinmd.com/blog/2014/03/assure-patients-side.html. Published March 28, 2014.

Gunderman, Richard, The Root of Physician Burnout. *The Atlantic*, August 27, 2012.

Harvard T. H. Chan School of Public Health, Who Mentored You: Maya Angelou. https://sites.sph.harvard.edu/wmy/celebrities/maya-angelou.

Jung, Carl Gustav, *Contributions to Analytical Psychology*, Harcourt Brace, New York, 1928.

Jung, Carl Gustav, Quotable Quote, Good reads. n.d. https://www.goodreads.com/quotes/50795-i-am-not-what-happened-to-me-i-am-what.

Kaplan, Karen. Cancer Survivors in the US—14.5 million strong and growing. *Los Angeles Times*, June 3, 2014.

KevinMD.com, About KevinMD.com, Kevin Pho, MD. https://www.kevinmd.com/blog/about-kevin-md. Accessed January 12, 2018.

King, Dr. Martin Luther, Jr., statement made in Chicago on March 25, 1966, to the second convention of the Medical Committee for Human Rights.

Kizer, Carolyn, Medicine, in *Cool, Calm, and Collected: Poems 1960–2000*, Copper Canyon Press, 2002, pp. 213–214.

Kornfield, Jack, *The Wise Heart: A Guide to the Universal Teachings of Buddhist Psychology*, Bantam Dell, Division of Random House, New York, 2008.

Kornfield, Jack, *A Lamp in the Darkness: Illuminating the Path Through Difficult Times*, Sounds True, Boulder, CO, 2011.

Kornfield, Jack, Right Understanding, October 28, 2016. https://jackkornfield.com/right-understanding/.

Kornfield, Jack, and Feldman, Christina, editors, *Stories of the Spirit, Stories of the Heart: Parables of the Spiritual Path from Around the World*, Harper, San Francisco, 1991. Excerpt from *Desert Wisdom*, Yushi Nomura, Orbis Books, 2001, p. 17.

Krauter, Cheryl, *Surviving the Storm: A Workbook for Telling Your Cancer Story*, Oxford University Press, New York, 2017.

Kumas-Tan, Z., Beagan, B., Loppie, C., MacLeod, A., and Frank, B., Measures of Cultural Competence: Examining Hidden Assumptions. *Acad Med.* 2007;82(6):548–557.

Lambda Legal, When Health Care Isn't Caring: Transgender and Gender-Nonconforming People Results from Lambda Legal's Health Care Fairness Survey, Lambda Legal, New York, 2010. https://www.lambdalegal.org/sites/default/files/publications/downloads/whcic-insert_transgender-and-gender-nonconforming-people.pdf.

Leap, Edwin, MD, KevinMD.com, Hospital CEOs Please Listen to Your Doctors and Nurses, March 15, 2016. https://www.medpagetoday.com/blogs/kevinmd/56862. Updated October 17, 2016.

Linden, Anné, *Boundaries in Human Relationships: How to Be Separate and Connected*, Crown House, Bancyfelin, Wales, 2008.

Lorde, Audre, When the Silence Shatters: Post-Black Women's Truth and Reconciliation Commission, Reflections from a Testifier, Ericka Dixon, BWB

Community Organizer and BWTRC Testifier, August 23, 2016. https://www.goodreads.com/quotes/141138-the-fact-that-we-are-here-and-that-i-speak.

Lowery, Amy E., PhD, and Holland, Jimmie, MD, Screening Cancer Patients for Distress and Guidelines for Routine Implementation [Review]. *J Community Support Oncol.* 2011 Nov 1. https://www.mdedge.com/jcso/article/47002/practice-management/screening-cancer-patients-distress-guidelines-routine?channel=270.

Maher, Bill, in Humorous Cancer Quotes and Sayings, n.d. Cancer Is Not Funny website. http://www.cancerisnotfunny.com/quotes.html.

McKinley, Elizabeth D., MD, MPH, Under Toad Days: Surviving the Uncertainty of Cancer Recurrence. *Ann Intern Med.* 2000;133(6): 479–480.

McLeod, S. A. Humanism. Simply Psychology. https://www.simplypsychology.org/humanistic.html. Updated 2015.

Mead, Margaret, Margaret Mead Quotes, BrainyQuote. n.d. https://www.brainyquote.com/quotes/quotes/m/margaretme100502.

Miller, Merry N., MD, and Ramsey McGowen K., PhD, The Painful Truth: Physicians Are Not Invincible. *South Med J.* 2000;93(10):966–973. https://www.ncbi.nlm.nih.gov/pubmed/11147478.

Mukherjee, Siddhartha, MD, *The Laws of Medicine: Field Notes from an Uncertain Science,* Ted Books, Simon and Schuster, New York, 2015.

National Institute of Health, National Cancer Institute, Office of Cancer Survivorship. Statistics. https://cancercontrol.cancer.gov/ocs/statistics/statistics.html. Last updated October 17, 2016.

Nekhlyudov, Larissa, Ganz, Patricia A., Arora, Neeraj K., and Rowland, Julia H., Going Beyond Being Lost in Transition: A Decade of Progress in Cancer Survivorship. *J Clin Oncol.* 2017;35(18):1978–1981. http://ascopubs.org/doi/full/10.1200/JCO.2016.72.1373.

Nomura, Yoshi, Desert Fathers, in *Stories of the Spirit, Stories of the Heart: Parables of the Spiritual Path from Around the World,* edited by Christina Feldman and Jack Kornfield, Harper, San Francisco, 1991.

Nomura, Y., *Desert Wisdom,* Orbis Books, New York, 2001.

Nye, Naomi Shihab, Kindness, in *Words Under the Words: Selected Poems,* Eighth Mountain Press, Portland, OR, 1995, pp. 42–43. Copyright © 1995.

O'Daniel, Michelle, and Rosenstein, Alan H., Professional Communication and Team Collaboration, in *Patient Safety and Quality: An Evidence-Based Handbook for Nurses,* edited by Pamela G. Hughes, Agency for Healthcare Research and Quality, Rockville, MD, 2008, Chapter 33.

Pearl, Robert, MD, How Our Patients Make Us Better, KevinMD.com. https://www.kevinmd.com/blog/2016/06/patients-make-us-better.html. Published June 19, 2016.

Peckham, Carol. Medscape Lifestyle Report 2016: Bias and Burnout. https://www.medscape.com/slideshow/lifestyle-2016-overview-6007335. Published January 1, 13, 2016.

Remen, Rachel Naomi, MD, Some Thoughts on Healing. http://www.rachelremen.com/some-thoughts-on-healing. Published August 16, 2010.

Remen, Rachel Naomi, MD, The Power of Wholeness, January 11, 2013. http://www.rachelremen.com/the-power-of-wholeness/.

Rogers, Carl, Quotable Quote, Good Reads. n.d. http://www.goodreads.com/quotes/411730-i-m-not-perfect-but-i-m-enough.

Rowe, Rosemary, and Calnan, Michael, Trust Relations in Health Care—The New Agenda. *Eur J Public Health*. 2006;16(1):4–6. http://eurpub.oxfordjournals.org/content/16/1/4.

Rowling, J. K. *Harry Potter and the Goblet of Fire*. https://www.goodreads.com/quotes/701025-dark-times-lie-ahead-of-us-and-there-will-be.

Satoro, Ryunosuke, Ryunosuke Satoro Quotes, BrainyQuote. 2017. https://www.brainyquote.com/quotes/quotes/r/ryunosukes167565.html. Accessed April 18, 2017.

Schneider, Kirk J., Existential–Humanistic Theories, in *Essential Psychotherapies, Third Edition: Theory and Practice*, edited by Stanley B. Messer and Alan S. Gurman, Guilford Press, New York, 2013, pp. 261–294.

Schneider, Kirk J., and Krug, Orah, *Existential–Humanistic Therapy*, American Psychological Association, Washington, DC, December 2010.

Shanafelt, T. D., Boone, S., Tan, L., et al., Burnout and Satisfaction with Work-Life Balance Among US Physicians Relative to the General US Population. *Arch Intern Med*. 2012;172(18):1377–1385.

Spotswood, Beth, Doctors' Storytelling Evening the Right Kind of Medicine. *San Francisco Chronicle*, May 18, 2016. http://www.sfchronicle.com/entertainment/article/Doctors-storytelling-evening-the-right-kind-of-7644051.php.

Stone, John, MD, Gaudeamus Igitur, in *Apartment 8: New and Selected Poems*, LSU Press, Baton Rouge, LA, 2004.

Strayed, Cheryl, *Brave Enough,* Knopf, New York, 2015.

Sutcliffe, Kathleen M., PhD, Elizabeth Lewton, PhD, MPH, and Marilynn M. Rosenthal, PhD, Communication Failures: An Insidious Contributor to Medical Mishaps. *Acad Med*. 2004;79(2):192.

Tervalon, Melanie, MD, MPH, and Murray-Garcia, Jann, MD, MPH, Cultural Humility Versus Cultural Competence: A Critical Distinction in Defining Physician Training Outcomes in Multicultural Education. *J Health Care Poor Underserved*. 1998;9(2):117–125.

Tervalon, Melanie, MD, MPH, Cultural Humility Training of Trainers [Training handout, Every Child Counts programs, Alameda County, CA], 2015.

Tolkien, J. R. R., in *The Silmarillion.*, edited and published posthumously by Christopher Tolkien, Allen and Unwin, London, September 15, 1977. https://www.goodreads.com/quotes/518504-all-have-their-worth-and-each-contributes-to-the-worth

UCLA Center for Mindfulness. About MARC. n.d. http://marc.ucla.edu/about-marc.

Wakefield Research. Press release for Dignity Health, November 13, 2013.

Wallin, David J., PhD, *Attachment in Psychotherapy*, Guilford Press, New York, 2017.

Whyte, David, *Everything Is Waiting for You*, Many Rivers Press, Langley, WA, 2003.

Williams, David R., PhD, MPH, and Wyatt, Ronald, MD, Racial Bias in Health Care and Health: Challenges and Opportunities. *JAMA*. 2015;314(6):555–556. doi:10.1001/jama.2015.9260.

Withers, Bill, Lean on Me, from the record album *Still Bill*, Sussex Records, released April 21, 1972. Reprinted by permission of Hal Leonard, LLC

Wolf, Jason, PhD, Patient Experience: Driving Outcomes at the Heart of Healthcare. *Patient Experience J*. 2016;3(1):1–4.

Yeager, Katherine A., PhD, RN, and Bauer-Wu, Susan, PhD, RN, FAAN, Cultural Humility: Essential Foundation for Clinical Researchers. *Appl Nurs Res*. 2013;26(4). doi:10.1016/j.apnr.2013.06.008.

Index

References to figures and tables are indicated with an italicized *f* and *t*.

cancer survivorship, *xviii*
 patient-centered care in, *xx–xxi*
 psychotherapy, *xix–xx*
 themes of, 24, 39–41, 54–58
cancer survivorship care, *xiii*
cancer treatment, end of, *xiii*
care
 importance of caring, *xxii–xxiii*
 self-, *xxv–xxvii*, 137–38
 see also self-care
caregivers, relationship with patients, 109
Carver, Raymond, 130
Center for Disease Control and Prevention (CDC), 18
Cheesecake Factory, business model, 34
Chodron, Pema, 102, 133
Chowdhury, Subir, 175
Chuang Tzu, 212
Cicero, Marcus Tullius, 184
Civil Rights Act (1964), 80
client-centered therapy, 5–6
clinical interview, basics of, 52–54
clinicians
 authentic interview with patients/clients, 52–54
 authentic listening, 33–35
 being authentic, 43–52
 being present, 45–46
 being with the challenges of work, 46–47
 bringing an open heart to work, 36–37
 burnout, 142–47
 cancer healthcare, 207–9
 collaboration in healthcare, 169–73
 community awareness, 73–76
 continuing to grow and develop, 50–51
 developing a disciplined sensitivity, 48–49
 finding meaning, 138, 147–50
 identifying with work, 51–52
 initial interviews, 130–31
 institutional awareness, 76–78
 interviewing patients and clients, 52–54
 learning cultural humility, 82
 mentoring, 173–74
 ongoing relationship with patients, 131–33
 relationship with patients, 96–97
 resources for, 211–12
 sacrificing self–care in service of patient, 166–69
 self-care, 138–42
 setting realistic personal standards, 51
 stories shared by, 189–94
 storytelling, 194–96
 stronger together, 175–76
 use of self, 44–52
collaboration
 clinicians stronger together, 175–76

clinicians supporting one another, 167–68
 common barriers to interprofessional, 165–66*t*
 practices building partnerships, 180–82
 questions for identifying meaning of, 177–80
 trust and dependence in healthcare, 169–73
 value of, 183–84
 workbook section, 177–84
Commission on Cancer, *xi*
communication
 common barriers to interprofessional, 165–66*t*
 four C's of, 38–39
 importance of caring, *xxii–xxiii*
 listening in, 33–35
 person-centered, in survivorship care, 33–36
 working with people, *xxvi–xxvii*
 skills in humanistic, workbook section, 42–60
community awareness, 73–76, 87
compassion
 questions for determining, 113–15
 in relationship, 102
 ways to develop, 115–16
concern
 clinical interview, 53–54
 in communication, 39
conversation, in communication, 39
Coulehan, Jack, 33, 139
Cripps, Amy, 141
cultural humility, 63–66
 approaching patients, 81–82
 breaking the silence, 79–80
 community awareness, 73–76, 87
 description of, 67–70
 developing awareness in, 83–89
 institutional awareness, 76–78, 88–89
 modes of learning, 82
 personal awareness, 70–72, 83–85
 professional awareness, 72–73, 85–86
 term, 64
 workbook section, 81–89
 see also humility
curiosity, in communication, 39

Darwin, Charles, 168
depression, cancer survivorship theme, 57
Dhand, Suneel, 24–25
distress screening, *xxiii*, 23
Doctors Who Create, 195
Doidge, Norman, 110
Dostoevsky, Fodor, 7

education, survivorship plan, 27–28
empathy
 definition of, 101

questions for determining, 111–12
  in relationship, 101–2, 111–13
  ways to develop, 113
Endgame (Beckett), 3
Epstein, David, 6
Erikson, Joan Serson, 106
ethnocentrism, 79–80
existential humanistic perspective
  being mindful of ourselves and others, 19–21
  in survivorship care, 12–13
existential humanistic psychotherapy, 3–6
Existential Humanistic Psychotherapy (Schneider and Krug), 6–7
existential humanistic therapy
  history of origins and foundation of, 6–11
  narrative interview, *xxiv–xxv*
Existential Humanistic–Therapy (Schneider and Krug), *xxii*, 5, 13
existentialism, 6, 7

Faber, Carl, *xxiii*, 33, 195
Falby, Cassandra, 25, 76–78, 79, 193
families, relationship with patients, 109
finding meaning, 138, 147–50
Frankl, Victor, 7
freedom, 7
Fromm, Erich, 8
Frost, Robert, 42

Gallagher, Nora, *xxiv*
Gawande, Atul, 12, 34
Goleman, Daniel, 106
Goodman, Sandra G., 102
Greif, Jon, 35, 99, 168, 176
Grumet, Jordan, 20
Gunderman, Richard, 143

Harvard Global Health Institute, 144
Harvard T. H. Chan School of Public Health, 144
healing relationship, *xiii–xiv, xviii*
health care. *See* clinicians
Health Care Fairness Campaign, 75
Heidegger, Martin, 7, 8
hierarchy of needs, Maslow's, 8, 9*f*
HIV communities, *xvii*, 75–76
Holland, Jimmie, 97
Hospital Writing Workshop (Campo), *xvii*
humanism, 6–7, 10, 11, 20
humanistic psychology, 8
  influence of, 10–11
  mindfulness and, 11–12
Humanistic Psychology Program (HPP), 3

humanity, 11
  cancer care and, *xx, xxvii*
  of clinicians, 23, 54, 81, 101, 107, 139, 143
  narrative storytelling, 80
human potential movement, 9
humility
  cultural, 63–66
  personal awareness, 70–72
  see also cultural humility
humor
  questions to determine, 125–26
  in relationship, 106–7
  ways to develop, 127
Husserl, Edmund, 7, 8

identity struggles, cancer survivorship theme, 55–56
income and life expectancy, United States, 65
Institute for Poetic Medicine, 139
institutional awareness, 76–78, 88–89
intentions
  long-term, 158
  self-care, 156–58
  short-term, 157–58
International Psychosocial Oncology Society (IPOS), 73, 74, 212

James, William, 8
Jha, Ashish, 144
Jones, Cheryl, 79
Jourard, Sydney, 8
Journal of Clinical Oncology (journal), 208
Journal of the American Medical Association (*JAMA*) (journal), 64, 68
Jung, Carl, 7, 8, 147

Kabat-Zinn, Jon, 160
KevinMD.com, 20, 195
Kierkegaard, Soren, 7
kindness
  questions for determining, 116–17
  in relationship, 103
  ways to develop, 118
"Kindness" (Nye), 63
King, Martin Luther, Jr., 80
Kizer, Carolyn, 96
Kornfield, Jack, 4, 11, 89, 102, 149, 159, 160
Krauter, Cheryl, 158, 189–90
Krug, Orah T., *xxii*, 5, 7, 13

Lamba Legal, survey by, 75, 90n.12
A Lamp in the Darkness (Kornfield), 11
The Laws of Medicine (Mukherjee), 23

trust
  collaboration among clinicians, 169–73
  questions for determining, 118–19
  in relationship, 104
  ways to develop, 119–20

UCLA Center for Mindfulness, 12
uncertainty, cancer survivorship theme, 24, 55
United States, association between income and life
    expectancy in, 65
University of California at Irvine, 64
University of California at Los Angeles (UCLA), 12, 63
University of California San Francisco, 194
University of Toronto Quality of Life Research
    Institute, 156–57

Verghese, Abraham, 194

Wakefield Research for Dignity Health, 103
Wallin, David, 97
"When the Silence Shatters" (Lorde), 66
White, Michael, 6
Whyte, David, 160, 177
The Wise Heart (Kornfield), 102, 149, 159
Withers, Bill, 169

Wolf, Jason, 110
Women's Cancer Resource Center, 66, 72, 76, 193
workbook section
  authentic clinician, 43–52
  authentic interview of patients/clients, 52–54
  clinical interview, 129–30
  collaboration, 177–84
  cultural humility, 81–89
  essentials of healing relationship in survivorship
      care, 111–29
  helping patients tell their stories, 58–60
  humanistic communication skills, 42–60
  initial interview and relationship, 130–31
  ongoing relationship, 131–33
  personal story, 197–203
  relationship, 110–33
  self-care, 151–60
  survivorship care, 29–31
  survivorship themes, 24, 39–41, 54–58
work-life balance, *xxvi*, 29

Yeager, Katherine A., 67, 71
Yoga for Healthy Aging, 159

Zen Buddhist tradition, 73